Anti-Inflammatory Diet for Beginners

The 3-Week Meal Plan to Naturally Restore the Immune System and Heal Inflammation with 84 Proven Easy Recipes

Steven Cole

Table of Contents

Introduction

Congratulations on downloading *The Anti-Inflammatory Diet for Beginners: The 3 Week Meal Plan to Naturally Restore the Immune System and Heal Inflammation with 84 Proven Easy Recipes* and thank you for doing so.

No matter if you are suffering from chronic inflammation or if you want to lead a healthier lifestyle, this book is for you! Throughout the pages of this book, you will find information to help you embark upon your anti-inflammatory diet journey. The transition from unhealthy eating to healthy eating may feel daunting at first, but rest assured that this book has you covered. As you read, remember that the transition to an anti-inflammatory diet is a lifestyle change, not a fad diet or a temporary fix.

In Chapter 1, we will discuss what inflammation is and examine different types of chronic inflammation diseases. In Chapter 2, we will discuss the benefits of why you should follow the anti-inflammatory diet and how it can heal your body. This chapter will also look at how to jumpstart your progress by kicking unhealthy habits. In chapters 3 and 4, we will discuss the types of food to avoid on this diet and what types of food you should eat, respectively. Chapter 6 will walk you through how to maintain an active lifestyle while eating the anti-inflammatory way. In Chapter 7, how to adjust to your new anti-inflammatory lifestyle will be the topic of discussion. Finally, in chapters 8 and 9, we will look at the three- week meal plan followed by 84 easy recipes to prepare.

There are plenty of books on this subject on the market, so thanks again for choosing this one! Every effort was made to ensure it is full of as much useful information as possible. Please enjoy!

Chapter 1: What Are Chronic Inflammation Diseases?

To better understand what an anti-inflammatory diet is, it is best to understand what inflammation is and how it affects our body. This chapter will cover the different types of inflammation, how they affect our body, and then examine a few diseases that are the results of chronic inflammation.

What is inflammation?

Inflammation is a natural body process. It is an important aspect, and oftentimes, the first step your body must take towards healing itself. There are two types of inflammation - acute and chronic. Inherently, short-term or acute inflammation is not a bad thing. Without acute inflammation, our bodies would not even heal. Acute inflammation is often the first step in the process of your body fighting against sickness or injury. This type of inflammation is a form of innate immunity, which means the way your body naturally protects itself against disease. Acute inflammation has a certain way of showing itself in our bodies when it affects the skin only. An acronym to identify this type of short-term inflammation is called PRISH.

- P - The 'P' in PRISH stands for pain. This means that the area that has inflammation is often painful to touch.

Other words to describe this type of pain can be 'throbbing,' 'stiffness', 'agonizing' or 'unbearable.'

- R - The 'R' means redness or discoloration. This normally occurs when blood rushes to the inflamed area.

- I - Immobility is what the 'I' means. The inflamed area is often unable to move or be of any use once inflammation occurs.

- S - The 'S' means swelling. When inflammation occurs, swelling or a building of fluid in the area can happen.

- H - Lastly, the 'H' stands for heat. Since more blood is flowing to the area where the inflammation is occurring, the affected area can become hot to the touch.

Acute inflammation typically lasts a few days until the affected area feels better showing that your body has successfully removed the threat to your body. However, when acute inflammation does not end, your body moves into long-term inflammation territory. So what are some of the causes of chronic inflammation?

Chronic inflammation can be the result of your body not successfully healing from an autoimmune disease. An autoimmune disease is one in which the body begins to attack itself. If the body is unable to heal, then it will be stuck in the inflammation stage which can cause consistent inflammation. If you are constantly surrounded by toxins in your body that affect you negatively, chronic inflammation can also occur. Think about if your body has ever had a negative reaction to paint or food? If you keep being around the issue that causes the allergic reaction, the issue will continue to occur. The same thing happens with chronic inflammation. If the environmental toxin is not removed, then your body will consistently have chronic inflammation. Lastly, chronic inflammation can occur if your body does not get rid of a pathogen that is causing illness. Unlike acute inflammation, if you are suffering from chronic inflammation, the results may not even show, especially if the inflammation is occurring deep inside your body, but similar to acute inflammation, there are some painful symptoms associated with chronic inflammation such as pain, heat, swelling, stiffness, and discomfort. But chronic inflammation also manifests itself differently in your body compared to acute inflammation. The danger with chronic inflammation is that if it never goes away, it can develop into serious, sometimes, life-threatening diseases within your body.

Some questions to determine if you are suffering from chronic inflammation include, "Are you obese?"; "Do you smoke?"; "Are you sleeping well at night?"; Are you having stomach issues or bloody stool?"; "Are you stressed in your everyday life?" If you said yes to one or more of these questions, you may be suffering from chronic inflammation. However, the best way to determine if you are suffering from chronic inflammation is to reach out to a doctor who will run a few tests to conclude if inflammation is the issue or not. These tests require that your blood is drawn. Then the blood is tested to see if you have certain proteins or markers in your blood that show you are suffering from chronic inflammation.

The common types of tests used to test chronic inflammation are an IL-6 test, a homocysteine test, C-reactive protein or (CRP) test, and the TNF alpha test. All of the tests are administered as blood tests when your blood is draw and then tested. An IL-6, or interleukin-6, is a protein found in your body when it has chronic inflammation. Homocysteine is also a type of amino acid found in the bloodstream. When you have a high level of IL-6 or homocysteine in your bloodstream, it could mean you are suffering from inflammation. C-reactive protein or (CRP) is also found in your bloodstream and produced by your liver. If you have high levels of this protein, it could point to inflammation. The TNF alpha test is the protein that your body automatically releases to your body's cells when you're sick which tells your body to start inflammation, so your body can begin the healing process. If you have a lot of this protein, it also means that you are testing positive for chronic inflammation. Depending on what type of chronic inflammation you have and which body part is affected will determine what type of treatment is needed. Unfortunately, many times, doctors do not know why your body is stuck in the inflammation stage. Chronic inflammation can be a result of genetics, illnesses or environmental toxins.

Chronic inflammatory diseases

This next section will explore some of the common illnesses that occur from the results of chronic inflammation.

Asthma

Asthma is caused by the chronic inflammation of your air passageways that carry oxygen to your lungs. Since this passage is inflamed, it causes one to have trouble breathing easily. Symptoms can be coughing, shortness of breath, wheezing, and chest tightening.

Rheumatoid arthritis

When your body begins to attack healthy tissues and inflammation results, this is called rheumatoid arthritis. The more your body attacks your tissue, the more severe the damage to your joints can be. Common body areas that are affected include your hands, feet, shoulders, and knees, but it can happen to any body part. Symptoms typically include swelling, loss of function in the affected area, and stiffness to name a few. This illness is one that doctors are unsure of why it happens. They usually prescribe medication, occupational therapy or surgery to treat.

Inflammatory bowel disease

When your digestive tract has inflammation, that disease is called inflammatory bowel disease which is the general term to describe it. Crohn's disease and colitis are two common types. A disease that is a direct effect of your digestive tract inflaming is called Crohn's disease. Colitis attacks the deep parts of your colon and can cause ulcers in your colon and rectum. Symptoms can include dramatic weight loss, diarrhea, fever, bloody stool, and cramping. Treatment includes medication and surgery.

Psoriasis

Psoriasis is the rapid build-up of skin cells and the inflammation that occurs when this happens. The built-up skin can become scaly, crack, and bleed. Psoriasis is not contagious and normally occurs on your face, scalp, hands, and feet, although, it can occur anywhere. It can be treated with lifestyle changes and medication

Hashimoto's disease

If your body and immune system negatively affect your thyroid, and it inflames, you can potentially have Hashimoto's disease. Initially, you may not notice any symptoms which cause it to get worse over time if you do not detect it quickly. Symptoms include feeling sluggish, swelling in your neck, unexplained weight gain, brittle nails, a pale face, memory lapses, and depression. Another major indicator is if you have an enlarged tongue. If you are suffering from any of this, it is best to see a doctor as soon as possible. This disease can be treated with hormones or alternative medicine.

Eosinophilic esophagitis

This disease is the inflammation of the esophagus. It is extremely rare and most people think they are suffering from heartburn. Other symptoms include issues with swallowing, vomiting or chest pain. The only way to test for it is to have a biopsy by a doctor.

Lupus

Lupus occurs when your body attacks its own tissues and organs. One of the most identifiable symptoms of lupus is a butterfly rash that develops across your face. Other symptoms include photosensitivity, headaches, joint pain, fever, and if your fingers and toes turn white or blue. To confirm if you have lupus or not, you must also be tested at a doctor's office.

Other well-known chronic inflammatory diseases include diabetes and heart disease. Scientists even think that inflammation plays a role in cancer, multiple sclerosis, and Alzheimer's disease. While medication and invasive surgeries can help the person deal with chronic illnesses, all can be treated by changing your diet to include foods that do not cause inflammation. Still not sure if a dietary change can affect your inflammation? Keep reading. The next chapter address this claim.

Chapter 2: The Benefits of Eating Smarter

With its focus on eating whole food, nutrient-heavy, and plant-based foods that prevent inflammation in the attempt to stop chronic inflammation, there are many other great benefits to the anti-inflammatory diet. In this chapter, the five benefits of eating an anti-inflammatory diet will be discussed.

The first benefit of the anti-inflammatory diet is weight loss. Due to the similar principles of eating more vegetables and fruit and limiting red meat like the Dash Diet and the Mediterranean diet, you can lose weight with the anti-inflammatory diet. Unlike the two diets, weight loss is not the primary motivator of embarking upon the anti-inflammatory diet. Weight loss is a welcome benefit. You lose weight with the anti-inflammatory diet because there are no caloric restrictions. The focus is on maximizing the types of healthy foods that you eat and listening to your body. As a result, your body will let you know when your full and you end up losing weight. When you lose weight, your inflammation also goes down. Since obesity is a major indicator of chronic inflammation when you lose weight, your chronic inflammation is automatically improved as well. Not just your inflammation, but the risk for other chronic inflammatory diseases like heart disease and diabetes also improve, too, since you are no longer overweight and limiting your salt and sugar intake.

The next benefit of the anti-inflammatory diet is an improvement of leaky gut. When the food you eat moves through your digestive tract, the nutrients from the food is processed into your bloodstream through tiny gaps in the intestines. These tiny gaps can loosen over time. If you are eating unhealthy foods, the nutrients that are being passed through can be marked as dangerous by your body, causing your body to attack itself and cause inflammation. If you are eating only healthy foods with awesome nutrients, leaky gut and your chronic inflammation improve concurrently.

Another major benefit of the anti-inflammatory diet is the money that you can save! Many chronic diseases are treated with expensive medications such as hormones and NSAIDs, or Non-steroidal Anti-Inflammatory Drugs. If you do not have good health insurance to cover the cost of this medication, you could be paying out from your pocket a lot. However, if you follow the anti-inflammatory diet, you treat your chronic inflammation at the root with your diet! Since you are already buying groceries, you are essentially saving yourself money by not having to buy expensive medication. You are also cutting down the cost of your grocery bill. When you buy healthy food, especially fruits and vegetables, they are usually cheaper than meat. With the anti-inflammatory diet's focus on healthy food, you can end up saving money and your health at the same time.

The most important benefit of the anti-inflammatory diet is the responsibility it stimulates on the person who practices it and the ability to share your info with others. Most people feel like there is no hope for their chronic inflammation, especially since doctors are oftentimes unable to figure out why it is happening in the first place. Consequently, some people wallow in their illness and do not take proactive precautions to improve their health. The anti-inflammatory diet puts you in the driver's seat of improving your health by something very effective which is your diet. You are able to fine-tune your health based on the food you like and what affect you. The doctor is not with you at every meal, but you are. You are able to figure out which foods trigger your inflammation through the process of elimination. You will be able to help others by sharing the information about which foods have helped your chronic inflammation.

Once you begin focusing on the lifestyle change that is the anti-inflammatory diet, you will notice the domino effect that it has on other aspects of your life. For example, you will begin to have a lot more energy. So what does that mean? You no longer need that cup of coffee or energy drink to sustain your energy. You also will be able to save money from not buying alcohol which is something that is not condoned with the anti-inflammatory dietary change. Your night's sleep will be so much more peaceful and amazing. You no longer must toss and turn at night, but the food you eat will help you have a more restful sleep. Not only just a restful sleep but you will be able to wake up in the morning without the use of an alarm clock feeling more energetic and less groggy. And that will directly translate to how the rest of your day goes.

Then once you notice the difference in your diet, you will be motivated to begin exercising if you aren't already doing so which will also improve your chronic inflammation. Next thing you know, your chronic inflammation has begun to get better, and it started by using your food as medicine! In the next two chapters, we will look at which foods are best to avoid and best to eat in the anti-inflammatory diet.

Chapter 3: Types of Food to Avoid and Why

Chapter 3 is all about which foods to avoid while on the anti-inflammatory diet. There are lots of foods that do not help with your chronic inflammation. This chapter highlights them, even the sneaky ones you may not notice in food that you are eating every day.

Alcohol overworks your liver. The anti-inflammatory advises that you drink as little alcohol as possible. This prevents your liver from having to work overtime which causes internal inflammation.

Sugar is a tricky product to avoid because it is usually in everything that we eat! When you eat sugar, it releases cytokines or proteins in your body that trigger inflammation. When looking for sugar, pay close attention to words that end in the three letters 'ose.' High Fructose syrup is a very important word to look out for! Junk food like cookies and sodas are very important to limit.

Aspartame is an FDA-approved product that is an artificial sweetener that gives you no nutrients in your body. Many people react negatively to it. If your body reacts negatively towards this product, it will cause inflammation since your body recognizes it as a foreign product. When you are looking for sugar in products that you are buying, be sure to watch out for aspartame. Good luck since it is in over 4,000 products!

White flour is found in white potatoes and rice, bread, crackers and rolls, French fries and instant mash potatoes. When you eat white flour products, they release advanced glycation. End products in these can cause inflammation. To prevent inflammation, it is best to avoid these products.

Processed foods are foods that are already prepared and require limited cooking. Foods in this category include soups and sauces in cans, pre-cooked freezer meat, microwavable dinners, and deli meat. These foods typically contain a lot of sugar, salt, and trans-fats. Avoid heavily processed foods, like microwavable dinners, packaged deli meats, and high-sodium canned soups and sauces. These foods are likely to contain added trans-fats, sodium, and sugars.

Omega-6 fatty acids are a necessity of your body to go through the natural growth and development cycle. In order for the natural growth and development cycle to be successful, your body needs a normal balance of fatty acids that are omega-3 and omega-6. When you eat too much omega-6 fatty acids, it throws your balance off and triggers inflammation in your body. The issue is that omega-6 fatty acids are found everywhere! They are in lots of salad dressings, mayonnaise, and most cooking oils. A major way to avoid omega-6 is to give up fried food which is found in lots of fast food.

Mono-sodium glutamate (MSG) is typically found in soup mixes, salad dressings, deli meats in Asian Foods, and soy sauce. This additive affects your liver's health and causes chronic inflammation. Try to avoid it.

Trans fats and partially hydrogenated oils are the same thing. Trans fats raise your LDL cholesterol (low-density lipoprotein cholesterol) levels. Too much LDL cholesterol can cause inflammation of your heart and heart disease. Do not buy it at all if you want to remain inflammation free.

Saturated fats can cause heart disease and make your arthritis inflammation worse! Saturated fats cause inflammation of your fat tissue. Guess what the biggest sources of saturated fats are? It is pizza and cheese! You can also get saturated fats from red meat. If you must have meat, choose the leanest cuts like sirloin, loin or ground. Then trim off as much fat as you can before cooking. Also, for the cheese and dairy lovers, go for low-fat dairy.

Salt can cause tissue inflammation! It is found in lots of junk food and many people tend to over salt their food. When you are cooking, try to use other herbs and spices besides salt to season your food and watch your inflammation go down.

Gluten is found in whole grains like barley, rye, wheat or casein. It is also found in some dairy products. For those that have arthritis, eliminating gluten can be helpful. If you notice that when you eat gluten, you have inflammation and pain, you could also be at risk for celiac disease. Once you give up gluten, you can determine if it is a trigger for your inflammation. Then proceed based on your results. If gluten does not bother you, feel free to eat whole grains. However, to take your anti-inflammatory diet to the next level, you can replace your whole grains with high-quality carbs like carrots squash and sweet potatoes.

In the next chapter, we will discuss all the good foods that you should eat!

Chapter 4: Types of Foods and Drinks to Eat

Finally! We get to talk about the good stuff, literally. In this chapter, we will discuss all the foods and drinks you can eat on the anti-inflammatory diet and why they are good for you.

Omega-3 fatty acids are responsible for building and growing your body. They are a good source of fatty acids to have. Omega-3 curbs inflammation. You can find Omega 3 and sausage like olive oil, walnuts, pumpkin seeds, hemp seeds, chia, and flax seeds. Algal oil is a great supplement to take to increase your omega- 3 fatty acids in your diet as well.

Other great sources of omega-3 fatty acids are fish that is super oily and super fatty like fatty sardines, mackerel, tuna, and salmon. When possible, opt for the wild version of fish and not the farm ones for more intense results.

Dark leafy plants that help stop inflammation are broccoli, red cabbage, spinach, kale, asparagus, and rainbow swiss chard. They are good sources of vitamin K which help with your chronic inflammatory diseases. You can even throw in collards which contain vitamin E. Vitamin E protects your cells from substances that want to cause inflammation. To take it to the next level, even try spirulina, celery, and chlorella which can lower cholesterol, too.

Blueberries, strawberries, blackberries, oranges, cherries, and raspberries all contain polyphenols which prevent inflammation. If you are ever craving sugar, they're all so great to have because they are low in sugar. These berries are also a good source of quercetin which fights inflammation and can even help prevent cancer. Also, do not forget about the acai berry which is another great food to have.

Maca is a great hormone regulator. This is often taken as a powder and it has lots of anti-inflammatory characteristics. Try to make it a staple in your diet like having it in or putting it in a smoothie.

Ginger is great for those suffering from arthritis especially osteoarthritis and rheumatoid arthritis and migraine headaches. The active component in ginger known as 6 - gingerol 1 is one of the major properties that prevent inflammation.

Turmeric's active property called curcumin exemplifies many anti-inflammatory characteristics. It is great for arthritis, diabetes, and cancer. Because turmeric can be difficult for the body to absorb, a lot of people try to take it, in fact, to help ease absorption. The more turmeric your body can absorb, the more it can help you prevent inflammation. If you are concerned about the yellow staining turmeric when you cook, you can opt for a curcumin supplement instead.

Sweet-potatoes and butternut squash plus other foods rich in beta-carotene are excellent sources of inflammation-fighting properties.

Cacao is best added to a smoothie, and if you want the sugar version, opt for dark chocolate. Cacao has over 300 compounds that help prevent inflammation. Do not forget about this wonderful food in your anti-inflammatory diet meal plans.

Coffee contains polyphenols which help prevent inflammation. To get the most out of coffee, try to choose a lighter roast and be sure to brew your coffee without a coffee filter. The best part about having coffee in your diet is it does not have to be caffeinated. A decaf cup of coffee contains just as many polyphenols as a caffeinated cup of coffee. If you do not like coffee at all, then you want to check out green or white tea because they contain just as many polyphenols. Green and white tea also contain catechins, another powerful property that fights inflammation.

Pineapple is another grapefruit to have because of bromelain. Bromelain helps your body prevent unnecessary inflammation. It also contains vitamin B1, potassium, magnesium, and vitamin C.

Beans have lots of fiber which is an important nutrient in fighting inflammation. Any type of bean is good for you, and it prevents inflammation!

Bone broth contains minerals that your body can absorb like magnesium, silicon, phosphorus, sulfur, and calcium which all help reduce joint pain arthritis and inflammation.

Whole grains like brown rice whole wheat bread and unrefined grains and oatmeal contain lots of fiber which can help your inflammation. If you do not have gluten sensitivity, feel free to eat whole grains but watch how much you eat to prevent unwanted weight.

Nuts, like walnuts, almonds, and cashews, etc., contain healthy fat that stops inflammation. Avocados, coconut, and olive oil are also good sources of healthy fats. These fats prevent unwanted weight gain as well. Celery also prevents inflammation and fights bacterial infections. It is an excellent source of potassium, as well as antioxidants and vitamins.

Water is an excellent source of hydration! It helps to flush toxins out your system that can cause inflammation. So drink up! Drink as much water as you can.

We've laid the groundwork for all sorts of food that you can eat on an anti-inflammatory diet. We will discuss recipes a little later in Chapter 8.

Chapter 5: Get the Most Out Of Your Food: How To Mindfully Purchase, Prepare, and Pair Foods for Maximum Nutrition

This chapter focuses on how to get the most out of your food in order to get maximum benefits from an anti-inflammatory diet. We will discuss how to find the best foods, how to prepare them, and how to pair them to get the maximum nutrition.

To make sure that you are getting the healthiest groceries for your anti-inflammatory diet, you may want to get organic products. But what does that mean? Organs mean that the plants were not exposed to radiation and do not contain any genetically modified organisms. It also means that it wasn't grown with any forbidden pesticides, sewage water or fake fertilizers. It also means that the animals with this sticker were farmed naturally with basic welfare and health standards. No antibiotics and growth hormones were given either, and the animal had access to outdoors. It also means that over 90% of the product is organic. If a product is organic, it will have a seal from the USDA. It usually costs farms lots of money to be able to put the USDA sticker on their products.

Other organic labels to check out are:

1. Free range which means that for poultry products, the birds had outdoors access.
2. Natural means the products have no artificial ingredients. However, there is no official meaning for 'natural' so companies can define this however they please.
3. Cage-free means that hens are kept in a setting where they can stretch their wings, nest, and walk, but they do not have to have access to outdoors. Forced molting by starvation and beak clipping can happen to these products.
4. Certified Humane means that the animals were comfortable for most of their lives and they are killed as painlessly as possible.
5. Fairtrade is normally a label for countries that are developing. The farmers had a working wage and decent work conditions.
6. Certified naturally grown products are essentially the same as USDA products, but not under USDA's jurisdiction for making sure that the USDA rules are enforced.

Organic product's produce sticker has five numbers and it begins with the number 9. Non-organic produce product sticker number, or the PLU code, only has 4-digits and the PLU code is only a total of 4 numbers. Some companies will use organic language on their produce, but not organic at all! Be sure to double-check. Also, there isn't an organic label for seafood as of yet, so you need to buy it organic. Just try to avoid fish that can contain high mercury levels like tilapia, sole, and oysters.

Produce that you will want to buy organic since they contain the highest level of pesticides are strawberries, apples, celery, potatoes, snap peas, cherry tomatoes, cucumber, bell peppers, grapes, spinach, nectarines, and peaches.

The cleanest produce from pesticides are eggplant, kiwi, cauliflower, sweet potato, pineapple, cabbage, frozen peas, onion, asparagus, mango, avocado, papaya, grapefruit, and sweet corn. These shouldn't have a priority to be bought organic. Foods that have to be peeled like bananas or oranges are also not as important to buy organic since you only eat the inside, not the outside. Lastly, quinoa has built-in natural pesticides that do not affect humans so there is no need to buy this one organic either.

Now that you know what produce to buy organically, where should you buy organic products? It is ideal to go to any local grocery store, but that can be expensive. To try and cut down the cost on your organic product, you can try to find a coop where you pay a yearly price and have access to healthy products all year long. You can also try to buy at a farmer's market or directly from a local farmer. Some farmers grow their food organically but are unable to pay for the USDA organic label, but you can ask them directly about their farming practices. Buying locally and in-season is also helpful on the anti-inflammatory diet. To try and find local farmers in the area, you can visit localharvest.org. Another cool trick is to try and buy non-perishable items online which can help cut down the costs or even try to grow some of the produce you use the most on your own.

How to Prepare Food

When you prepare your anti-inflammatory diet, there are a few other great practices to keep in mind.

- Instead of using salt, try to use different spices like cilantro, garlic or turmeric, all of which contain anti-inflammatory properties.

- You can also try to use cinnamon or nutmeg instead of sugar.

- When searing food, try to use water instead of oil.

- If you are not sure if the produce is good or not, just throw it out.

- Also, try to use cooking methods that are better than frying like steaming, roasting, grilling or boiling them.

Try to avoid oils and butter when you are cooking your vegetables.

- To avoid cross-contamination, keep the raw food and cooked food's utensils separate. Also, do not make hot foods cold or cold foods hot unnecessarily.

- Wash your product with light salt and water to cleanse all the dirt way.

Awesome Food Pairings

When you cook certain foods together, it boosts the healthiness of the produce and ensures you are getting the maximum inflammation busting qualities of the food. What are these food-pairings, you say?

Here they are:

Sodium and potassium. Sodium brings the nutrients to your body while potassium washes away what you do not need. Our typical diet doesn't contain a lot of potassium so if you eat more, that's helpful. A great source of potassium is celery. Potassium also pairs well with magnesium. A pair like beets and broccoli is a good one to have.

Magnesium and calcium. Too much calcium can cause inflammation and painful kidney stones. By pairing the calcium with magnesium, it balances out the calcium to prevent unnecessary inflammation.

Spicy foods and beta-Carotene used together help increase the absorption of Vitamin A which helps you with your inflammation. For example, you can put pepper or chili powder on sweet potatoes or butternut squash to help your body absorb more Vitamin A and ward off inflammation.

Vegetables and healthy fat. A vegetable and healthy fat pairing increase the absorption of lutein and beta-carotene in your system. This duo joins together to fight inflammation. An example would be to put olive oil over your next salad.

Probiotic plus probiotic. An example of this would be kefir and your favorite type of nut. This helps fight off chronic inflammation in your intestines.

Two other great pairings would be Quercetin and Ellagic Acid found in raspberries and grapes, then combining iron-rich foods and citruses like lentils and lemons. Both of these pairing form super combos that help you fight inflammation.

Chapter 6: How to Uphold an Active Lifestyle on the Anti-Inflammatory Diet

Chapter 6 discusses how to maintain an active lifestyle while on the anti-inflammatory diet. Here's a little secret. Exercise causes inflammation. Hear me out. When you do a tough workout, your body initiates acute inflammation to repair and rebuild your cells. However, this type of acute inflammation is good in the short-term which results in helping you improve chronic inflammation. If you notice that you are constantly tired after doing an intense workout, this point to you potentially having chronic inflammation. You may want to consider altering your exercise routine, doing shorter periods or change your workout to see if your chronic inflammation persists or not. The most important thing when working out is to make sure that you are recovering between your workouts in order to get the most out of your exercise regimen.

Some types of exercises that are really good to couple with your anti-inflammatory diet and boot the diet's benefits are yoga, walking or hiking.

Yoga is so great at fighting inflammation because of the deep breathing. When oxygen goes to your cells, it repairs them quickly and helps with chronic inflammation. The deep breathing associated with doing yoga is an excellent inflammation buster. There are three poses that are very helpful with combating inflammation that we will discuss, but any restorative yoga pose is beneficial to preventing inflammation.

Half lord of the fish is the first pose. This reduces chronic inflammation by cleaning the digestive system and organs associated with your intestines. To start, you find a comfortable place to sit and extend both of your legs. You put the right foot outside the left quad as far as possible. Then you put your foot on the left side outside the hip on your right side. Then you want to swing the elbow on your left side of your body to the knee on the right side of your body. Try to get it as far to the outside of your right knee as you can. You can use the hand on your right side as extra support. Now in this pose, you want to be mindful of your back. Make sure that you are listening to your spine by drawing the crown of your head to the sky. You want to try this on both sides and then hold 5-7 deeps breaths on each side.

The next pose that's really helpful to reduce inflammation is called the bridge pose. To do the bridge pose, you lie on your back and bend your knees. Then place both feet parallel to the floor. Put both hands close to both hips and put your palms parallel to the floor with your palms downward. You want to breathe in and lift your hips and try to bring your chest as close as possible to your chin. You want to keep your core strong and have one long line from your knees to your shoulders. Again, hold your breath for 5 to 7 breaths on each side for maximum benefits.

Another very popular yoga pose to battle chronic inflammation is called the child's pose. You first want to get comfortable by doing the tabletop pose which is simply putting your shoulders and your wrist forwards then putting your hips over your knees. You want to bring your big toes as close as possible. Then you want to gently sit on your hip. This allows the Torso to rest between your knees with your arms stretched out in front of you as far as possible. Hold for 5 to 7 breaths on each side as well.

The next exercise that is great for reducing inflammation is simply walking. Do not underestimate walking's power to fight inflammation. Walking is so great at reducing inflammation because it sends fresh oxygen and blood throughout your body. In turn, this helps clean out your digestion and combat inflammation. After a very tough workout, walking is great to reset your system and prepare you for your next workout. To take your walking to the next level, go for a hike. Immersing yourself in nature helps lower your cortisol stress response, that is very important in reducing inflammation. Overall, no matter, what exercise you do, it is important to listen to your body. It will tell you when it had enough or if you should keep going.

After your workout, it is important to make sure that you are eating an anti-inflammatory meal with foods that will help you recover after doing a workout. After working out, if you can reduce inflammation, it will help prevent the soreness that comes up sometimes after your workout called delayed onset muscle soreness or DOMS. Eating about 30 to 60 minutes after you cool down will help replace the glycogen stores that will help you heal quickly. Some great foods to eat after working out would be black beans because they help repair muscle damage. Leafy greens like spinach, Brussel sprouts, kale, broccoli are another good food to aid in your post-workout recovery. They help you hydrate without causing a spike in sugar. If you are pressed for time and do not have time to make a meal, a quick and easy post-workout snack is to add spices to yogurt or in a post-workout smoothie like turmeric, ginger or cinnamon.

And what about carbs you say? No worries. The best carbs to eat after a workout would be whole-grain carbs that have lots of fiber. When you have fiber-rich foods, it can lower the inflammatory c-reactive protein which is a marker for inflammation. Some of the best whole-grain carbs to have are brown rice, bulgur, quinoa or oatmeal.

Another tip to prevent anti-inflammation after a workout is to do a workout right when you wake up if it is cardio. This helps your inflammation and helps you burn more weight since your body is already in a caloric deficit from the night before. If you are doing weight training, you may want to eat a little something about 30 to 60 minutes before so you can digest your food before the workout. For cardio, a banana or fruit smoothie about 30 minutes beforehand is great. For weight training, you may want to try something a little heavier like whole-grain pancakes about 3-4 hours before the workout.

After your workout, no matter if it is cardio or weight-training, try to avoid sports drinks as they have lots of sugar. Also, you want to drink as much water as possible. Most importantly, do not eat too much after your workout or before your workout so you negate the workout that you do.

Caloric Maintenance

So exactly how many calories do you need to burn to have a great workout? That's totally up to you. A weight-loss workout is totally different than if you are trying to maintain weight. One of the easiest ways to figure out how much weight you are burning is to use a calorie counter. A simple app can be on your phone like MyFitnessPal, Lose It! or My Diet Coach.

A rule of thumb is that if you want to lose weight, you calculate that by using this formula: All of your burned calories = Length of workout (not seconds, convert to minutes) x (3.5 X your weight in kilograms x Metabolic Equivalent (or MET)) divided by two hundred.

It takes 3,500 calories to lose 1 pound of weight so if you want to lose 20 pounds you have to multiply 20 * 3500 for a total of 70,000 calories in order to lose the weight. If you do not want to calculate it manually, you can use any calorie calculator online that's free like healthstatus.com. However, if you want to calculate it manually, know that MET stands for Metabolic Equivalent. Here are a few MET values of the common activities that we do.

Light Activities	Value
Waking very slow	2.3
Desk work	1.5
Watching TV	1.0
Sleeping	0.9
Moderate Activities	
Sexual Activity	5.8
Home exercise	3.5
Walking moderately	3.3
Bicycling lightly	3.0
Intense Activities	
Jumping Rope	10.0
Heavy home exercises	8.0
Jogging	7.0

Nutrient Timing

Knowing when to eat foods is very important when following the anti-inflammatory diet. It helps you prevent discomfort and aids in digestion. Also, be mindful what you are eating based on your activity level. Ultimately, these are guidelines to follow and you should do best according to how your body responds.

Breakfast

To make sure you get all your vegetables, you can eat a savory, vegetable-based breakfast so that you get what you need. Really, vegetables are great to have at any time of day because they help stabilize our mood, especially if you get stressed throughout the day.

Avoid oranges at breakfast because it can cause stomach irritation which can lead to inflammation.

Avoid zucchini for breakfast because it has a diuretic effect and can cause dehydration if you haven't drunk anything yet for the morning.

The best time to eat apples is at breakfast because of the pectin in the apple's skin. Pectin helps your intestines remove toxic things from your body. Apples are horrible at dinnertime because apples increase stomach acid which can lead to discomfort.

Tomatoes are great to have at breakfast because the type of acid found in tomatoes can help your digestive processes and regulate the functions of your stomach and pancreas.

The best time to have potatoes is at breakfast because it lowers our blood cholesterol level and it is also rich in minerals that your body needs to power you throughout the day.

A fiber-packed bowl of oatmeal, topped with peanut butter and berries sets the tone for the day for your digestive tract.

Also, have chocolate for breakfast. Sounds counterintuitive, but when you have dark chocolate in the morning, it protects your skin against sun rays and it gives you all day to burn the calories off.

Lunch

The best time to eat carbohydrates is during and after physical activity because this is when your body can best handle them. You may want to eat a lower amount of carbs daily if you are sedentary most of the time to prevent weight gain.

The best time to eat meat is at lunchtime. It helps to reduce fatigue by giving a steady flow of nutrients throughout the rest of the day. It also takes meat about 5 hours to digest. By eating it at lunch, you give your body ample time to digest the meat. However, if you eat meat at dinner, be sure to eat it early enough before you go to bed so your food can be digested.

Another great thing to eat at lunch is raw nuts because it helps your body with the fatty acids that are omega-3. Since nuts have a high-calorie count and fat count, if you eat them for dinner, you can gain unwanted weight.

Pasta is best to have for breakfast and lunch so your body can digest the food throughout the rest of the day.

The best time to have rice is at lunch as it is high in carbohydrates and can help you stay energized. If you eat rice at dinner, then it could potentially lead to weight gain.

Dinner

Because potatoes are two to three times higher in calories than other vegetables, you do not want to have them for dinner.

Tomatoes at dinnertime can cause swelling.

For dinner, it is great to have something spicy to aid in digestion, but if you have an unfavorable reaction, please avoid.

Chapter 7: Tips on Transitioning to an Anti-Inflammatory Lifestyle

When you transition to the anti-inflammatory diet, you will need the inspiration to keep going when the tough times come! When you want that ice cream or that bag of crispy chips, but you know you are focusing on being healthy, the tips in this chapter will help you maintain your new healthy lifestyle and conquer those cravings that you are having.

The first tip to keep in mind is to have an anti-inflammatory vision board with a pictorial representation of your goals for going on the anti-inflammatory diet. You can use magazines, newspapers, or coupons, or a simple hand-drawn explanation to keep your goals right in front of you. During a moment of weakness, a quick glance to your board may be the trick to help you keep going. You could also use social media to pinpoint your favorite anti-inflammatory practitioners and blogs that you can check out when you want inspiration.

You will also want to consider keeping a food journal. It is a cool way to track your progress and to celebrate your victories. You can get an old notepad or a journal and keep daily track of what you ate during the day, making notes if you had any cravings, and did you give in or how did you handle it? A food journal will help you note patterns in your diet and what works for you and what doesn't in order to help you maintain the anti-inflammatory lifestyle as successfully as possible.

Make a personal goal to share your journey with someone else. Sharing your journey with others can add more meaning to it, and it can help others see the benefits of living an anti-inflammatory lifestyle.

As you transition, remember to take baby steps. You did not get chronic inflammation overnight, so you should also not expect it to heal overnight. Do not expect to lose 50 pounds in one week. Keep your goals realistic and celebrate your small successes. Remember, this is not a diet, this is a lifestyle. As long as you are staying true to the lifestyle, the results should come. Remember to keep going, do not stop, and let the diet do the work for you.

Think about why you are eating or snacking? This may help you stop eating things that aren't good for you.

If you make a mistake, do not get discouraged. Tomorrow is a new day. Treat it like that and get back on your anti-inflammatory horse and ride it.

Host a dinner party! This will help others see what you are doing and help you on your journey.

Learn the anti-inflammatory equivalent of your favorite recipes from your desserts to your favorite pasta. Also, look for healthy substitutions of what you like.

A serving is equal to one cup of raw food or half a cup when it is cooked. A great rule of thumb is to try and eat 9 servings of fruits and vegetables every day.

Try at least one recipe or one new spice a week. This will help keep your journey fresh and fun. Also, never stop learning. Keep researching and learning about the anti-inflammatory diet so you can keep getting great results.

If you like to snack, try to eat at least 2 snacks daily. You can take anti-inflammatory supplements like fish oil or curcumin at that time as well.

Be prepared! Try to pre-cook your meals, so when you are feeling hungry you will not slide since you already have food prepared. You can also keep little snacks in places that you always visit so you have access to easy snacks.

If you do not like something or a tip doesn't work for you, do not feel guilty for not doing it. An anti-inflammatory diet is one that you can modify and you can adjust to your liking.

Get into the habits of reading ingredient lists. This can help you spot inflammatory ingredients that you didn't know where there. You can also double-check your sauces and condiments as well to see if they are causing inflammation or not.

Drink water! Drinking lots of water help you stay hydrated and can be extremely helpful.

Lastly, eat as many vegetables and healthy anti-inflammatory foods as you can? When was the last time you heard someone say that they got sick from eating so many vegetables?

Chapter 8: 3-Week Meal Plan

Week 1:

	Breakfast	Lunch	Dinner
Sunday	Overnight oats with blueberries and a cup of green tea	Loaded baked sweet potato and a side of zucchini noodles and chopped vegetables	Lentil veggie bowl with Brussel sprouts, broccoli, and sweet potatoes
Monday	Cinnamon quinoa breakfast bowl	Large mixed green salad with an egg on top drizzled with olive oil	Veggie burger with a lettuce bun, small salad, and carrot fries
Tuesday	Raspberry smoothie	Lemon and herb sardine salad with an apple	Salmon patties, broccoli, and a green salad
Wednesday	Pineapple	Chickpea	Shrimp and

	ginger smoothie with protein powder	Vegetable coconut curry with steamed rice	vegetable curry
Thursday	Spinach, Kale, Banana smoothie	Cauliflower steak with beans and tomatoes	Vegetable and sweet potato hash with a slice of avocado
Friday	Chia overnight pudding with strawberries and raspberries	Lettuce wraps with smoked trout and a side of cauliflower rice	Buddha bowl with 3 steamed veggies, 1 protein, & 1 carbohydrate of your choice with your favorite dipping sauce
Saturday	Steel cut oats topped with blackberries	Quinoa stuffed green and red peppers	Tuna burgers with sweet potato buns and a side salad
Sunday	Breakfast	Grilled	Rainbow salad

	Salad of mixed greens and a fried egg on top	salmon asparagus and green beans	with every color of veggie and fruit

Week 2:

	Breakfast	Lunch	Dinner
Sunday	Ezekiel bread with scrambled eggs and turmeric	Quinoa, spinach and citrus salad	Stir-fry chicken with green and red peppers
Monday	Avocado, mango and apple smoothie	Curried tofu and cabbage	Quinoa taco bowl with spinach, peppers, beans, tomatoes and avocadoes
Tuesday	Overnight peanut butter chia seed pudding	Black beans, brown rice and plantain	Zucchini sushi with carrots, avocado and cucumber

Wednesday	Sweet potato frittata	Grilled sardines on toast with mashed avocado	Cucumber and melon salad
Thursday	Mini quiche, broccoli and salsa cups	Eggplant parmesan and wheat pasta	Spinach, tomato, and zucchini noodle spaghetti
Friday	Pineapple Oatmeal	Loaded veggie, baked sweet potato	Roasted buffalo cauliflower lettuce wraps
Saturday	Blueberry French Toast Sticks	Salmon burgers	Orange chicken, couscous and a mixed side salad
Sunday	Apple cinnamon pancakes	Salad in a jar with all of your favorite topping	Spicy butternut squash soup

Week 3:

	Breakfast	Lunch	Dinner
Sunday	Apple cinnamon pancakes	Hummus and cucumber sandwich	Chicken tacos
Monday	Tofu tostadas with turmeric	Lean beef stew	Grilled vegetable skewers and cauliflower and broccoli rice
Tuesday	Biscuits, turkey bacon, and Jam	Sardine, tomato and mixed greens sandwich	Chicken, zucchini noodle soup
Wednesday	Trout and quinoa with your favorite hot sauce	Soy and ginger chicken wings	Stuffed peppers Mexican style
Thursday	Apple muffins	Pear and carrot salad	Scrambled tofu (like turkey meat), broccoli and

			sweet potatoes
Friday	Rice cakes, peanut butter and honey	Orange and cranberry smoothie	Lettuce and pea soup
Saturday	Oatmeal, peanut butter and chia seeds breakfast cookies	Curry chicken in the slow cooker served with rice	Pita pizza and a side of julienned veggies
Sunday	Avocado toast and mixed cherry tomatoes	White bean, cabbage and kale quesadillas	Tikka Masala Chickpeas served over spinach

Chapter 9: 84 Easy Recipes

The point of this chapter is to give 84 quick recipes for the more experienced cook. Enjoy.

Breakfast

Simple Chia Pudding

This recipe takes about 6 hours and 5 minutes to prepare and makes 4 servings.

The serving size is 0.5 g. It contains:

- 6.9 grams Protein
- 3 grams Sugar
- 9.5 grams Fiber
- 16.3 grams Carbohydrates
- 23 milligrams Sodium
- 4.3 grams Saturated fats
- 10.3 grams Fat

What to Use

- Extract (Vanilla) (1 teaspoon)

- Agave (1-2 tablespoons)
- Dairy-free milk (1.5 cups)
- Seeds - Chia (0.5 c)

What to Do

1. First, combine the maple syrup, vanilla extract, chia seeds, and dairy-free milk in a bowl. Then whisk the ingredients very well to mix them all together.

2. Refrigerate the ingredients overnight or for at least 6 hours in the bowl (preferably overnight) so the chia pudding is thick and creamy. If the chia pudding is not thick and creamy, you can add more chia seeds. Then put it back into the refrigerator, and keep it in the refrigerator for about another hour or so until the pudding is firm. You can garnish it with fruit or almonds or nuts of your choice.

Baked Eggs

This recipe takes about 10 minutes to prepare and cook for four servings.

The serving size is two eggs, and it contains:

- 400 milligrams Cholesterol
- 13 grams Protein
- 204 milligrams Sodium
- 1 gram Sugar
- 1 gram Carbohydrates
- 9 Saturated fats
- 19 grams Total fat

What to Use

- Toasted bread (for serving)
- Salt and Pepper (to taste)
- Unsalted butter (2 tbsp)
- Heavy cream (low-fat or vegan option for a healthier choice) (2 tbsp)
- Large eggs (8)
- Cheese (Grated, and Low-fat or vegan) (1 tbsp)
- Parsley (1 tbsp)
- Rosemary (smidget)
- Thyme (smidget)

- Fresh garlic (smidget)

What to Do

1. Pre-heat your oven broiler for 5 minutes, putting below the heat about 6 inches in the oven rack.
2. Next, mix the cheese and herbs.
3. Then crack two eggs in four individual small bowls without breaking the yolk. You will not be baking the eggs in this dish so be careful to avoid breaking the yolk.
4. Put the 4 individual baking ramekins on a baking sheet. Put a 0.5 tbsp of cream and butter in each ramekin, putting each one 3 minutes in the broiler until the mixture is hot and bubbling.
5. When it's bubbling, take the ramekin out of the oven. Carefully and very slowly pour two eggs into each ramekin.
6. Then sprinkle the herb mixture, salt, and pepper in each ramekin. Put the small dishes back into the oven until only the whites of the eggs are nearly finished. Remember, eggs will cook when you take them out the oven so try not to overcook.
7. Serve with the toasted bread of your choice.

Powerful Anti-inflammatory Smoothie

This recipe takes 10 minutes to make and makes two servings.

A serving is a cup, and it contains:

- 4 grams Protein
- 53 grams Carbohydrates
- 50 milligrams Sodium
- 15 milligrams cholesterol
- 3 grams Saturated Fat
- 5 grams Total fat

What to Use

- Low-fat vanilla frozen yogurt (1 c)
- Honey (1 tbsp)
- Lime juice (3 to 4 tbsp)
- Chilled brewed green tea (0.5 c)
- Frozen chopped peeled mangoes (1-1.5 c)

What to Do

1. Combine all the ingredients into a powerful blender, except the frozen yogurt, and blend until all the

ingredients are combined. Then add frozen yogurt and blend until smooth.

2. You can also substitute almond milk or non-dairy milk for the yogurt. You can also substitute green tea too.

Berry Smoothie Bowl

This recipe takes 5 minutes to make and it makes one serving.

A serving is one bowl and it contains

- 2.8 grams Protein
- 25.9 grams Sugar
- 8.8 grams Fiber
- 47.5 grams Carbohydrates
- 9 milligrams Sodium
- 1.6 grams Saturated fat
- 2.5 grand total

What to Use

- Protein powder (1 scoop)
- Almond milk (2-3 tbsp (can substitute coconut milk))
- Sliced ripe banana (1 that is frozen)
- Organic Frozen mixed berries (1 big c)
- Seeds (Hemp and Chia) (1 tbsp)
- Shreds of coconut (Unsweetened) (1 tbsp)

What to Do

1. Blend the berries and ripened banana together.

2. Add the almond milk to the protein powder and blend both until the mixture is blended smoothly. You can top with chia seeds, hemp seeds, or shredded unsweetened coconut if you would like.

3. You can also substitute any non-diary milk if you do not like dairy milk. To take the recipe to another level, you can also substitute a green or white tea as well.

Sweet Potato Kale Hash

This recipe takes 10 minutes of getting it ready, 35 minutes to cook it all, and makes 2 servings.

A serving contains:

- 15.7 grams Protein
- 9 grams Sugar
- 6.8 grams Fiber
- 37.3 grams Carbohydrates
- 911 milligrams Sodium
- 12.8 grams Saturated fats
- 18.8 grams Total fat

What to Use

- Kale bundle (1 large one)
- Ground turmeric (0.125 teaspoon)
- Fresh parsley (2 tablespoons)
- Red onion (1)
- Salt and pepper (0.5 teaspoon each)
- Coconut sugar (1 teaspoon)
- Tandoori Masala spice (3.25 teaspoon)
- Melted coconut oil (2 tablespoon)
- Sweet potatoes (2 small ones)
- Extra-firm tofu (8 oz package)

- Pre-heat your oven to 400 degrees Fahrenheit. Before you make the tofu, you want to get it as dry as possible so it will crisp up nicely and be extra crispy.

- To dry out the tofu, take the tofu out of the package and put the tofu in a clean towel. Then put a skillet or pot on the towel that is on top of the tofu so it can squeeze out the extra moisture. If the towel becomes soaking wet while following this step, you can replace it with another clean towel.

- While the tofu is drying, chop the sweet potatoes into small cubes and season them. Next, slice the onions and season them as well. Then, combine the onions and potatoes onto a lightly greased baking pan.

- Bake the potatoes and onions for 25 to 35 minutes and flip them one time while cooking so both sides can be nice and brown.

- You will know they are finished cooking when the onions are caramelized and brown and the sweet potatoes are tender. Remove the potatoes and onions from the oven. Put them in another bowl so they won't keep cooking on the tray, and set them to the side.

- While the potatoes and onions are cooling, put the dried out tofu in a bowl and scramble it well with two forks. The tofu should be scrambled into small pieces, and they will look like scrambled eggs somewhat.

- Then, in your large skillet, heat the cooking oil, add all your spices, and sauté your tofu for 5 minutes. You want to get the tofu as brown and dry as possible without burning it. Set the finished tofu aside.
- In the same pan, put a little extra oil and sauté your kale, followed by adding your tofu back in. Divide the kale, sweet potatoes, onion, and tofu into bowls equally and serve.
- You can serve with a hummus or a hot sauce.

Cantaloupe Boats

This recipe takes 15 minutes to prepare, and it makes 1 serving.

A serving contains:

- 13.8 grams Protein
- 13 grams Fiber
- 79 grams Carbohydrates
- 34 milligrams Sodium
- 4.3 grams Saturated Fat
- 16 grams Total Fat

What to Use

- Granola
- Hemp Seeds (0.5 tablespoon)
- Chia Seeds (1 tablespoon)
- Sliced Almonds (2-3 tablespoons)
- Blueberries (0.25 cup)
- Cherries (0.5 cup)
- Kiwi (1 medium one)
- Dairy-free yogurt (1 cup)
- Ripe cantaloupe (halved with seeds removed)
- Agave (optional)

- Cinnamon (optional)

What to Do

1. First, the cantaloupe boats need to be scooped out. Scoop the insides out and then leave a little flesh about 1-2 inches.
2. Then fill the cantaloupe boats by adding the yogurt, fruit, nuts, and seeds to the inside.
3. You can also drizzle with agave or honey. You can also sprinkle a little cinnamon on the top.
4. Save the insides to add to a smoothie for later.

Sweet Potato Toast

This recipe takes 5 minutes of preparing time, cooking time at 10 minutes, and creates 4 servings.

The serving size is a 0.25-inch thick slice, and it contains:

- 0.5 grams Protein
- 1 grams Fiber
- 1.4 grams Sugar
- 17.9 grams Sodium

What to Use

- 1 sweet potato
- Maple syrup or honey
- Cinnamon (optional)
- Ginger (optional)
- Your favorite nut butter (optional)

What to Do

1. Carefully slice the sweet potato into four slices that are 0.25 inches thick.
2. Then, insert a 'slice' into the toaster. Test this toaster out to see which settings are the best settings so you can 'toast' the other potato toast slices. Let the potato slices

toast until they are tender with a few browned spots on the potato. Be careful that you do not burn them.

3. When they are ready, you can pop them out and then garnish them.

4. You can then drizzle honey or maple syrup on top. Then even add a little ginger for extra benefits. You can also choose to sprinkle with your favorite nut butter, like almond or peanut and sprinkle a little cinnamon on top.

Frozen Citrus Cups

This recipe takes 60 minutes to prepare, 3 hours or longer to freeze, and it makes 90 servings.

A serving is 1 cup, and it contains:

- 1 gram Protein
- 11 grams Sugar
- 11 milligrams Sodium

What to Use

- Large firm bananas (5 sliced)
- Frozen orange juice concentrate (5 cans slightly thawed)
- Mandarin oranges (5 11 oz cans drained)
- Unsweetened pineapple tidbits (5 cans, 20 oz each)
- 10 cups boiling water
- Lemon gelatin (5, 3 oz packages)

What to Do

1. Put a pot of water on and let it boil.
2. Then add the gelatin to the boiling water. Then mix in the remaining ingredients. Let it cool down enough so you will not burn yourself.

3. Get your cupcake pan and then put muffin liners on the inside of it.

4. Put the gelatin mixture and the fruit into the foil cups inside your muffin pan. Then place the whole tin back into the fridge's freezer or stand-alone freezer, and keep it in there for about 3 hours or longer until the mixture is frozen.

5. When you are ready to serve the citrus cups, take out the citrus cups 30 minutes before serving.

6. You can serve with Greek yogurt, dairy-free yogurt or by themselves.

Breakfast Patties

This recipe takes 30 minutes to prepare, and it makes 16 patties.

A serving is 1 patty, and it contains:

- 10 grams Protein
- 275 milligrams Sodium
- 5 gram Total fat

What to Use

- Pepper (Cayenne) (0.5 tsp)
- Ginger (Ground) (0.5 tsp)
- Pepper (Black) (1 tsp)
- Leaves (Dried Sage) (1 tsp)
- Salt (Kosher or Pink) (1.5 tsp)
- Lean ground turkey (2 lbs)

What to Do

1. Stir all the various ingredients in a mixing bowl. Then shape your ingredients into sixteen 2.5 inches separate patties.
2. Then fry them about 5 minutes until there is no pink left.

3. You can eat by itself or serve with any type of leafy green like kale, swiss chard, collards or arugula.

Three Ingredient Pancakes

This recipe takes preparation time of 5 minutes, cooking time 15 minutes for 16 portions.

A serving is one pancake, and it contains:

- 2 grams Protein
- 2 grams Sugar
- 1 grams Fiber
- 6 grams Carbohydrates
- 101 milligrams Potassium
- 28 milligrams Sodium
- 1 grams Total fat

What to Use

- Coconut flour (0.3 c)
- Eggs (6)
- Bananas (3 large ripe ones)
- Honey or Agave (optional)
- Cinnamon (optional)
- Extra-virgin olive oil or coconut oil (for frying)

1. Blend everything and mix them. If you need to smooth the mixture out, you can add your favorite non-dairy milk. If it gets too runny, you can add more flour, a tablespoon at a time.
2. Once your batter is ready, go ahead and put a little oil in your pan for frying.
3. Then fry the pancakes for about 120 seconds.
4. You can garnish with the toppings of your choice like honey, chia seeds, hemp seeds, fruit, cinnamon, your favorite nut or your favorite non-dairy whipped cream.

Fast Blueberry Smoothie

This recipe takes 6 minutes to prepare, and it makes 2 servings.

A serving contains:

- 8 grams Protein
- 46 grams Sugar
- 4 grams Fiber
- 61 grams Carbohydrates
- 561 milligrams Potassium
- 34 milligrams Sodium

What to Use

- Vanilla Greek Yogurt (0.75 c)
- Frozen Blueberries (1.5 c)
- Banana (1 cut into two pieces)
- Apple, white grape, or almond milk (1.5 c)
- Extra fruit (raspberries, blueberries, apple slices, your choice for garnish)
- Almonds (optional)
- Cinnamon (optional)
- Ginger (optional)

What to Do

1. Blend all ingredients in a powerful blend until they are the consistency that you want.
2. You can garnish with nuts, fruit, almond or a dash of cinnamon or ginger.

Quick Acai Bowl

This recipe takes preparation time of 10 minutes, and it makes 2 servings.

A serving contains:

- 1 grams Fiber
- 6 grams Protein
- 43 g Carbohydrates
- 387 mg Potassium
- 33 grams Sugar
- 23 mg Sodium

What to Use

- Toppings of your choice (chia seeds, coconut, sliced bananas or berries)
- Acai Berry puree (1 3.5 oz frozen packet)
- Honey (1 tbsp)
- Vanilla Greek yogurt (0.5 c)
- Frozen Berries (1.5 c)
- Banana (1 sliced)
- Apple juice (1 c)
- Almonds or your favorite nut (optional)

What to Do

1. Blend all ingredients until very smooth. Add liquid to thin the acai bowl out or add more fruit to make it thicker.
2. Top with the garnish of your choice.
3. Pour into a big bowl to eat.
4. To take the recipe to another level, add a dash of ground ginger or almonds. You can also use a white or green tea instead of apple juice.

Peanut Butter Overnight Oats

This recipe takes preparation time of 15 minutes, setting time of 6 hours, and creates one serving.

A serving contains:

- 14.6 grams Protein
- 14.9 grams Sugar
- 12 grams Fiber
- 50.9 grams Carbohydrates
- 162 milligrams Sodium
- 2 grams Saturated Fat
- 23.9 grams Total fat

What to Use

- Toppings of your choice (flaxseeds, chia seeds, granola, or berries)
- Oats (0.5 c)
- Maple Syrup (1 tbsp)
- Favorite Peanut Butter (2 tbsp, can be creamy or chunky)
- Chia seeds (0.75 tbsp)
- Unsweetened almond milk (0.5 c)

1. Add all the ingredients, except the oats, to a bowl or mason jar and mix them together. Make sure everything is mixed well to distribute it. If you do not want the peanut butter, you do not have to add the peanut butter.

2. Add the oats and stir the ingredients again. Make sure all the oats are submerged in the milk. If you need to add a little more liquid, you can to make it a little soupier if that is your preference.

3. Refrigerate the overnight oats for at least 6 hours. In the morning, put the toppings of your choice.

Fantastic Breakfast Salad

This recipe takes preparation time of 5 minutes, cooking time of 15 minutes, and it makes a single portion.

A serving contains:

- 29 g Total fat
- 3 g Sugar
- 17 g Protein
- 13 g Carbohydrates
- 7 g Fiber

What to Use

- Salt (to taste)
- Avocado (0.3 of the avocado and make it sliced)
- Roasted cauliflower (0.5 c)
- Baby greens of kale, spinach or your favorite (2-3 c)
- Chopped red onion (0.25 c)
- Eggs or egg substitute (1 to 3)
- Cooking oil of your choice (2 tsp)

1. Sauté the onions until they are soft in the extra-virgin olive oil.

2. Then add in the roasted cauliflower and greens to the skillet. Sprinkle with a salt. Put the mixture into a bowl.

3. Then add more oil to the skillet, and make the two eggs how you like it. Once the eggs are ready, put them on top of the salad.

4. You can add a little hot sauce and sprinkle with ginger to take it to another level.

Grapefruit Pineapple Detox Smoothie

This recipe takes preparation time of 10 minutes, and it makes 2 servings.

A serving contains:

- 4 grams Protein
- 28 grams Sugar
- 3 grams Fiber
- 37 grams Carbohydrates
- 7 grams Total fat

What to Use

- Fresh Ginger (0.25 inch, sliced)
- Coconut oil (1 tbsp)
- Greek yogurt (0.3 c)
- Pineapple chunks (2 c)
- Red grapefruit (1)
- Chia seeds (optional)
- Hempseeds (optional)
- Protein powder (optional)
- Cinnamon (optional)

1. Blend everything.
2. You can add extra grapefruit sections on top for a garnish.
3. You can add chia seeds or hemp seeds or protein powder for extra protein.
4. A little cinnamon on top of the smoothie will add extra benefits as well.

Pineapple Anti-inflammation Smooth

This recipe takes 5 minutes to prepare, and it makes 1 serving.

A serving contains:

- 4 grams Protein
- 28 grams Sugar
- 9 grams Fiber
- 43 grams Carbohydrates
- 11 grams Total fat

What to Use

- Fresh ginger (1 knob sliced)
- Lemon juice (1-2 tsp)
- Baby kale (1 c)
- Coconut water (0.75 c, can use regular water or light coconut water to make it healthier)
- Frozen pineapple (1 c)
- Apple (a half one chopped and cored)
- Unsweetened Apple juice (optional)
- Green or white tea (optional)

What to Do

1. Blend all ingredients until you get the desired consistency that you want.
2. If you want it to be slightly thicker, add yogurt instead of coconut water.
3. You can add more water, unsweetened apple juice, green or white tea to thin it out. You can also add agave juice as well.

Quinoa and Cinnamon Breakfast Bowl

This recipe takes preparation time of 5 minutes, cooking time of 15 minutes, and creates 2 portions.

A serving contains:

- 14 grams Protein
- 15 grams Sugar
- 8 grams Fiber
- 94 grams Carbohydrates
- 6 grams Total fat

What to Use

- Fresh fruit of your choice (2 c)
- Maple syrup (2 tbsp)
- Cacao nibs (2 tbsp)
- Salt (to taste)
- Extract (Vanilla) (0.5 tsp)
- Cinnamon (to taste)
- Milk (Non-dairy or dairy) (1 c)
- Water (Filtered or Purified) (1 c)
- Uncooked quinoa (1 c)

What to Do

1. When you begin, rinse the quinoa well and drain the excess water off. Place the quinoa to the side.
2. Then put the quinoa, water, and almond milk in a saucepan and boil it.
3. When the quinoa and the mixture starts boiling, reduce it to a simmer and season with the salt and taste of vanilla.
4. Turn off the heat when the liquid is gone. When it is finished, fluff the quinoa and top with the fruit, maple syrup, and cacao. Add more liquid to thin.

Breakfast Cookies

This recipe takes preparation time of 5 minutes, cooking time of 15 minutes, and it creates 12 portions.

A serving contains:

- 1.5 g Protein
- 67 g Fat
- 10.5 g Carbohydrates

What to Use

- Cinnamon (1 teaspoon)
- Quick Oats (1 c)
- Bananas (2)
- Honey or Agave (to drizzle)

What to Do

1. Before you begin, 350 degrees should be set on your oven.
2. Smush bananas and quick oats together in a bowl.
3. Stir all the ingredients well, then add 1 tsp of cinnamon and stir.
4. Scoop out a heaping tablespoon of the mixture on a greased baking sheet until all spots are filled.

5. Bake for a total time of 15 minutes.

6. When cool, you can eat hot and drizzle with honey. Or you can cool them and save it for later.

Pumpkin Spice Muffins

This recipe takes preparation time of 5 minutes, cooking time of 20 minutes, and it makes 12 servings.

A serving contains:

- 6 grams Protein
- 24 grams Sugar
- 8 grams Fiber
- 93 grams Carbohydrates
- 24 grams Total fat

What to Use

- Cake Mix (Spike Cake or Carrot) (1 15.25 oz box)
- Puree (Pumpkin) (1 15 oz can)

What to Do

1. Preheat the oven to 350 degrees before you take the next steps.
2. Get your muffin tin out. Then put muffin liners in the muffin tin.
3. Then mix the spice cake mix and pumpkin puree together. Do not over mix it.
4. Bake for 20-25 minutes.

5. When they are done, you can add yogurt on the top as an icing or eat them by itself.

Egg, Toast, and Turkey Bacon Cups

This recipe takes preparation time of 10 minutes, cooking time of 20 minutes, and makes 12 cups.

One serving contains:

- 10 grams Protein
- 11 grams Carbohydrates
- 8.5 grams Total fat

What to Use

- Eggs (12)
- Turkey Bacon Slices (12 cooked 75% of the way)
- Whole Wheat or Gluten Free Bread (12 slices)

What to Do

- Preheat the oven to 375 degrees. Before you start assembling the steps, go ahead and have your turkey bacon slices cooked at least 75%. The turkey bacon will finish cooking while in the cut.
- After you get the turkey bacon settled, go ahead and remove the crust from each side of the bread slices, and smash each piece of bread with a baking pin. Try to get it as flat as possible.

- Then cut a circle into the bread. Once the circle is cut, cut the circle diagonally.
- Spray a muffin tin well and place the diagonal halves in the muffin space. Be sure to not have any space showing on the bottom.
- Then cut the turkey bacon in half and place each one in an individual cup on each side of the muffin tin. You can have at least one half of the turkey bacon higher than the side. Once the bread and the turkey bacon are arranged, you can bring out the eggs.
- Break the eggs into each muffin space. You do not have to scramble them.
- Bake for at least 20 minutes or until the egg is to your preference.

Slow Cooker Cinnamon Apple Oatmeal

This recipe takes preparation time of 10 minutes, cooking time of 6 hours, and creates 4 portions.

A serving contains:

- 5 g Protein
- 4 g Fiber
- 3 g Sugar
- 4 g Total fat
- 26 g Carbohydrates

What to Use

- Dried fruit, chopped nuts, and/or sugar (for garnishing)
- Salt (to taste)
- Cinnamon (to taste)
- Vanilla (to taste)
- Agave (1 tbsp)
- Apples (1 cup chopped)
- Vanilla Almond milk (1.5 c)
- Water (2.5 c)
- Steel cut oats (1 c)
- Coconut oil (for spreading around the slow cooker)

- Put the coconut oil around the inside of your slow cooker. Add it liberally. If it is not coated fully, the ingredients will stick to the side of the crockpot.
- After the slow cooker is coved, you can add all of your ingredients together and mix them well.
- Put on the setting of low and cook at least 5-8 hours.
- When ready to serve, top the dish with the topping of your choice. You can add fruit, almonds or a nut of your choice.

Lunch

Simple Lentil Soup

This recipe takes preparation time of 15 minutes, cooking time of 20 minutes, and creates 7 cups.

The serving size is 1 cup, and it contains:

- 8 grams Protein
- 4 grams Sugar
- 8 grams Fiber
- 24 grams Carbohydrates
- 250 milligrams Sodium
- 11 grams Saturated fat

What to Use

- Fresh lime juice (2 tsp)
- Baby spinach (1 5 oz pack)
- Pepper (Cayenne) (to taste)
- Pepper and salt (according to taste)
- Low salt vegetable broth (3.5 c)
- Uncooked red lentils (0.75 c rinsed and cooked)
- Coconut milk (1 can, 15 oz)
- Tomatoes (Diced) (1 can, 15 oz)
- Ground cardamom (0.25 tsp)

- Cinnamon (0.5 tsp)
- Cumin (Ground) (1.5 tsp)
- Turmeric (Ground) (2 tsp)
- Garlic cloves (Minced) (2 large cloves)
- Onion (Diced) (2 c)
- Cooking oil (1.5 tbsp)

What to Do

1. Sauté the minced garlic cloves and diced onions within the large pot in the cooking oil for about 4 to 6 minutes over medium heat until the onion is soft. Put in the salt and fry it until it is fragrant.
2. Add ground cardamom, cinnamon, turmeric, and cumin and stir until combined well. Continue to cook for about one more minute until it smells nice.
3. Then add a full can of coconut milk and full can of diced tomatoes, including the juices. You can put in the cayenne pepper to taste if you feel like it.
4. Stir all the ingredients together until it is combined. Then increase heat until it reaches a low boil.
5. When it begins to boil, turn down the heat and let it cook until the lentils are tender.
6. Turn it off and add the spinach until it wilts. Add in the lime juice then decide if you want to add more salt and pepper.

7. You can serve with toasted bread of your choice, a leafy salad or vegetables. This recipe also holds up well in the refrigerator so you can prepare a huge batch and freeze it for later.

Carrot, Turmeric Ginger Smoothie

This recipe takes 25 minutes to prepare, and it makes 2 cups.

A serving is 0.5 cups, and it contains:

- 2.5 grams Protein
- 17.5 grams Sugar
- 5 g Fiber
- 32 g Carbohydrates
- 112 milligrams Sodium
- 2.3 grams Fat

What to Use

- Unsweetened almond milk (1 cup)
- Lemon juice (1 tablespoon)
- Carrot juice (2.5 cups)
- Ground turmeric (0.25 teaspoon)
- Fresh ginger (0.5 tablespoon)
- Pineapple (1 cup, can be fresh or frozen)
- Banana (1 ripe one)

1. Put everything in a very powerful blender. Blend all the ingredients until they are a smooth drink.

2. Adjust the flavors to your liking. You could also use your favorite agave or coconut juice, green or white to thin it out as well.

3. You can garnish with extra ginger, pineapple, carrot or turmeric. Watch out for the staining of the turmeric. To take it to the next level, you can add a dash of cayenne pepper.

Apple Carrot Ginger Beet Juice

This recipe takes preparation time of 10 minutes and makes 1 serving.

A serving contains:

- 41 g Sugar
- 6 g Fiber
- 3 g Protein
- 63 g Carbohydrates
- 209 mg Sodium
- 1 gram Fat

What to Use

- Carrots (3 whole ones)
- Fresh Ginger (1 tablespoon)
- Apple (1 medium one)
- Beet (1 medium one)

What to Do

1. Peel your fruit and veggies. Rinse them well. You can even wash it in a baking soda and water solution or a salt and water solution.

2. After the ingredients are clean, you can place them in a blender and blend them all together until all the ingredients are smooth or the consistency that you would like.

3. You can keep the pulp for extra benefits and add unsweetened apple juice to thin it out. You can add it to a salad or a smoothie. You could also use your favorite agave or coconut juice, green or white to thin it out as well.

4. You can garnish the juice with extra chopped garlic or thinly sliced carrots.

Avocado Toast

This recipe takes 5 minutes to prepare and makes 1 serving.

A serving contains:

- 14 grams Protein
- 3 grams Sugar
- 17 grams Fiber
- 43 grams Carbohydrates
- 977 milligrams Potassium
- 162 milligrams Sodium
- 6 grams MSG
- 5 grams Polyunsaturated fat
- 4 grams Saturated fat
- 24 grams Total Fat

What to Use

- Whole grain bread (2 slices)
- Hemp hearts (1 tablespoon)
- Radishes (2 thinly sliced)
- Lemon juice (1 tsp)
- Avocado (1 pitted and peeled)
- Cherry Tomatoes (optional)
- Peppers (optional)

- Apple (optional)
- Low-fat or vegan parmesan cheese (optional)

What to Do

1. Mash the avocado and lemon juice together until it forms a paste. If you do not like a lot of avocado chucks mashing. If you want to smooth it out, add a smidget more of lemon juice.
2. Once the avocado is the consistency that you want, you can spread half of it on one bread slice.
3. You can top it with radishes and garnish using salt or pepper or both together if desired.
4. Other ideas for garnish can be sweet mini peppers, cherry tomatoes or even slices of apple. You can also garnish with low-fat parmesan or vegan cheese.

Cold Cucumber Soup

This recipe takes 15 minutes to prepare and makes 4 servings

A serving contains:

- 1 gram Protein
- 6 grams Sugar
- 2 grams Fiber
- 11 grams Carbohydrates
- 122 milligrams Potassium
- 159 milligrams Sodium
- 1 gram Fat

What to Use

- Sliced almonds (to garnish)
- Diced red pepper and cucumber (to garnish)
- Salt (0.5 teaspoon)
- Lime juice from half a lime
- Apple (1 sweet one of your choice, cored and peeled)
- Green onion (2)
- Basil Leaves (5 fresh ones)
- Garlic cloves (2)
- Unsweetened Almond Milk (1 cup)
- English cucumbers (2 or about 4 cups)

- Broth (bone, chicken, beef, optional)
- Low-fat cheese (optional)

What to Do

1. Wash your produce well and then peel them. If they have seeds, you can remove them if you would like.
2. Once the produce is ready, you can chop them into small pieces and place it in a powerful blender.
3. Combine every ingredient together well. If you need to thin it out, you can add more water. You can also use a bone broth, like chicken or beef or vegetable instead of almond milk.
4. Once all the ingredients are blended according to the consistency you would like, you can chill the soup. You can also serve it slightly warm.
5. When you are ready to eat it, garnish with the toppings of your choice.
6. You can use fresh basil leaves or parsley or your favorite low-fat cheese.

Chickpea Salad

This recipe takes preparation time of 10 minutes and makes 3 servings.

A serving contains:

- 5 grams Fiber
- 4 g Sugar
- 7 g Protein
- 25 grams Carbohydrates
- 263 milligrams Potassium
- 31 milligrams Sodium
- 8 grams Total fat

What to Use

- Salt and Pepper (according to your taste)
- Seasoning (Poultry) (0.5 teaspoon)
- Dill that is dried (0.5 teaspoon)
- Dijon mustard (1 tablespoon)
- Vegan May like Just Mayo or Vegenaise (2 tablespoons)
- Sliced Grapes (0.5 cup)
- Green onions (2 chopped)
- Celery stalk (1 diced)
- Chickpeas (1 15 oz can)
- Crackers (for serving)

- Whole-grain (toast)
- Sprouted bread (toast)

What to Do

1. Before you begin, rinse and drain the chickpeas.
2. Empty the chickpeas into a small bowl and slightly mash the chickpeas with a fork. You can smash according to the consistency you want. The mixture can either be completely smooth or you can leave a few whole chickpeas in place throughout the mixture.
3. After the chickpeas are smashed according to your liking, add in the remaining ingredients and mix well. You can add a little more mayo if you are having issues mixing everything together.
4. When you are finished mixing everything together, put the mixture in the refrigerator until it is ready to serve with crackers or toasted whole-grain or sprouted bread.

Kale Apple Salad with a Hot Pumpkin Vinaigrette

This recipe takes preparation time of 10 minutes, cooking time of 3 minutes and makes 4 servings.

A serving contains:

- 6 s Protein
- 18 g Sugar
- 2 g Fiber
- 151 milligrams Potassium
- 30 g Carbohydrates
- 309 milligrams Sodium
- 9 grams MSG
- 4 grams Polysaturated Fat
- 2 grams Saturated Fat
- 15 grams Total fat

What to Use

Dressing

- Cooking oil (0.25 cup)
- Salt and pepper (according to your to taste)
- Shallots (1 teaspoon, minced)
- Agave or syrup (Maple) (1 tablespoon)
- Vinegar (Apple cider) (0.25 cup)

- Pure pumpkin puree (0.33 cup)

Salad

- Apples (sliced)
- Dried cranberries (0.25 cup)
- Shelled pumpkin seeds (0.33 cups)
- Pecans (0.33 cups)
- Kale (1 curly bundle, thinly chopped)

What to Do

1. Wash the product well.
2. Chop the vegetables well, too. Mix together the maple syrup or agave, minced shallots, salt, and pepper, pumpkin puree and vinegar in one small sauce pot. Then drizzle in the olive oil slowly. Heat on the stove to warm, and whisk the mixture often to prevent it from burning.
3. While the dress is warming up, combine all your salad ingredients in another bowl. Make sure is everything chopped according to the size that you want.
4. Once the dressing is warm, pour it over the salad.

Vegetable and Egg Bowl

This recipe takes 10 minutes to prepare, 25 minutes to cook, and makes 4 servings

A serving contains:

- 10 grams Fat
- 34 grams Carbs
- 11 grams Protein
- 8 grams Sugars

What to Use

- Sweet potatoes (1 lb)
- Brussels sprouts (1 lb)
- Apple cider vinegar (3 tbsp)
- Arugula (2 c)
- Harissa (tablespoon (3))
- Cooking oil (1.5 tbsp)
- Eggs (4)
- Hot Sauce (optional)
- Ground ginger (optional)

What to Do

1. Set your oven to 400 degrees.

2. As your oven is warming up, cut your Brussel sprouts in half. Then chop the sweet potatoes into small pieces.

3. After the vegetables are cut up, grab a baking tray and cover it in aluminum foil.

4. Pour olive oil over the vegetables and roast them for about 17-20 minutes.

5. Whisk the harissa with the extra-virgin olive oil and apple cider vinegar in a side bowl and put it to the side.

6. Then fry your eggs to your preference. You can mix a little ginger and salt and pepper in with the oil while you fry it. You can also poach them if you would like.

7. When the eggs are ready to serve, divide the Brussels sprouts and sweet potatoes and arugula amongst four bowls. Then drizzle the harissa sauce over it.

Carrots, Quinoa & Oranges Recipe

This recipe takes preparation time of 15 minutes, cooking time o f3.5 hours, and creates 4 servings.

A serving contains:

- 3 g Total Fat
- 1 g Saturated fat
- 31 g Carbohydrates
- 5 g Protein
- 230 mg Sodium
- 11 g Sugars
- 5 g Fiber

What to Use

- Salt and Pepper (to taste)
- Ground cardamom (a pinch)
- Ginger (one, 1-inch piece fresh and minced)
- Golden Raisins (0.3 c)
- Carrots (peeled and sliced)
- Bone broth (2.5 c)
- Quinoa (1 c rinsed well)
- Oranges (2)
- Extra-virgin olive oil

- To begin, go ahead and rinse and drain the quinoa. Put it to the side while you prepare the rest of the recipe.

- Coat the slow cooker with extra-virgin olive oil.
- Peel the oranges and carefully scrape away the white underside.
- Once you have the zest, peel the fruit from the oranges and zest the oranges.
- Then put the quinoa, broth, carrots, raisins, ginger, salt, black pepper, and orange zest in a slow cooker and stir well.
- Cook until the quinoa is tender which should take about 3 to 3.5 hours.
- Serve with the extra pieces of fruit over the top of it.

Grilled Avocado Sandwich with Sauerkraut

This recipe takes 10 minutes of prep time, cooking time of 12 minutes, and creates 4 servings.

A serving contains:

- 14 grams Fat
- 781 milligrams Sodium
- 552 milligrams Potassium
- 39 grams Carbohydrates
- 10 grams Protein

What to Use

- Whole-grain or sprouted bread of your choice (8 slices)
- Vegan or butter spread
- Hummus (1 c)
- Sauerkraut (1 c drained, rinsed lightly, and liquid squeezed out as much as possible)
- Avocado (1 big one peeled and sliced long ways into about 16 pieces)
- Low-fat cheese (optional)

1. Before you begin, start your oven to 400 degrees. Butter your bread and toast your slices.

2. When they are finished, spread the hummus over each slice.

3. Add the prepared sauerkraut and then add the avocado slices.

4. Take about half of the hummus and distribute over the 4 slices of bread then distribute the sauerkraut over the hummus on each slice. Add in the avocado slices over the sauerkraut.

5. You can bake the sandwiches a little bit longer until they are golden brown if you prefer.

6. To take this recipe to the next level, you can choose to add a little cheese as well and sprinkle it over the top.

Chilled Lemon Zucchini Noodles

This recipe takes 25 minutes to prepare, and it makes 4 servings.

A serving contains:

- 19 grams Fat
- 8 grams Carbs
- 2 grams Protein
- 5 grams Sugars

What to Use

- Salt and pepper (to taste)
- Lemon (1 zested and juiced)
- Mustard (Dijon) (0.5 teaspoon)
- Powder (Garlic) (0.5 tsp)
- Cooking oil (of your choice) (0.3 c)
- Zucchini (3 medium ones cut into noodles)
- Radishes (1 bunch thinly sliced)
- Thyme (1 tbsp chopped)
- Cauliflower florets (optional)
- Broccoli florets (optional)
- Low-fat or dairy-free cheese option (optional)

1. Combine the lemon zest and juice, powder garlic, and mustard in a small container. Whisk them all together.

2. Slowly add in cooking oil of your choice. Again, whisk it all and combine. Use salt and pepper to season it according to how your taste buds like it. When it is mixed well, you can go ahead and put it to the side to prepare the rest of the ingredients.

3. Wash the zucchini and you can peel it or decide not to. Once it is peeled or not, you can go ahead and cut them with a zoodler.

4. When the noodles are ready, in a large bowl, toss the zucchini noodles and radishes.

5. You can add in your dressing sitting in your bowl to the side and toss until the veggies are well coated.

6. Garnish with fresh thyme and serve. A modification to this recipe is you can add as many vegetables as you like. You can consider adding broccoli or cauliflower florets. You could even add chopped pepper as well. To take it to another level, you can choose to add a low-fat or dairy-free cheese option, too.

Caprese Tomato Salad

This recipe takes preparation time of 20 minutes and it makes 4 servings.

A serving contains:

- 2 g Fiber
- 4 g Sugar
- 2 g Protein
- 5 grams Carbohydrates
- 207 milligrams Sodium
- 5.8 gram Total fat
- 2.7 gram Monosaturated fat
- 0.4 gram Polysaturated
- 1.9 grams Saturated Fat

What to Use

- Fresh mozzarella cheese (1 oz low-fat or vegan and diced)
- Salt (according to your taste)
- Black Pepper (according to your taste)
- Vinegar (Balsamic) (1 tablespoon)
- Olive oil (Extra-virgin) (1 tablespoon)
- Leaves (Basil) (0.5 c)
- Cherry Tomatoes (3 cups halved)
- Whole-grain bread (optional)

- Sprouted bread (optional)
- Lettuce wraps (optional)

What to Do

1. Combine a pinch of salt and the tomatoes in a big bowl. Mix them all together to let the flavors fuse.
2. Let it stand for 5 minutes.
3. Then add in the basil leaves, balsamic vinegar, a pinch of salt and pepper, mozzarella, and toss. You can serve with fresh basil.
4. If you want to make the mixture into a sandwich, you can add the mixture to a lettuce wrap or on top of your favorite whole-grain or sprouted grain bread. Or you can enjoy it on its own.

Skirt Steak with Red Pepper and Corn

This recipe takes 1 hour and 10 minutes to prepare, and it makes 4 servings.

A serving contains:

- 18.2 g Total fat
- 19 g Carbohydrates
- 3 g Fiber
- 676 mg Sodium
- 10.4 grams MSG
- 1.6 g Polysaturated Fat
- 5.2 g Saturated Fat
- 25 g Protein
- 8 g Sugar

What to Use

- Salt and Pepper (to taste)
- Fresh corn kernels (2 cups from about 3-4 ears)
- Olive oil (2 tbsp)
- Water (1 c)
- Red bell peppers (divided into two)
- Skirt steak (1 lb)
- Green onions (0.75 c chopped and divided)
- Fish sauce (3 tbsp)

1. To begin this recipe, start off by making the marinade. Mix about 0.3 cups of the onion and fish sauce in a shallow bowl. Coat the steak. Let the steak stand at room temperature and then turn it in the bag after thirty minutes so the steak can be well-coated.

2. While the steak is marinating, cut the bell pepper into 1-inch pieces and combine with 0.25 c of onion in water. When it is finished, just so the onions are soft, you can blend them together in a powerful blender until they are smooth. Then stir in your salt and oil.

3. Slice your peppers and add your pepper slices and corn and the remaining onions to a cast iron skillet.

4. Cook until the peppers are wilted and the corn is slightly charred. Stir in 0.25 teaspoon of salt and black pepper. Remove it from the pan and keep it warm.

5. Then extract the steak out the marinade liquid and toss your marinade liquid out.

6. Then put the skillet on high heat and add the steak.

7. Cook on 3 minutes on both sides until the steak is glazed on both sides. You can also cook it to your liking at this stage.

8. Then cut the steak diagonally into slices and serve with the pepper and corn mixture. You can garnish with thyme if you want.

Roasted Chicken and Carrots in One Pan

This recipe takes preparation time of 15 minutes, cooking time of 20 minutes, and creates 4 servings.

A serving contains:

- 37 grams Protein
- 10 grams Sugar
- 39 grams Total fat

What to Use

- Rosemary (1 tbsp)
- Carrots (1.5 peeled and trimmed)
- Salt and Pepper (according to your taste)
- Extra-virgin olive Oil (four tbsp)
- Onion (1 cut and peeled into eights)
- Chicken thighs (4)

What to Do

1. Set your oven's heat to 425 degrees. Put your carrots and onion assembled by one single layer on a liberally greased baking sheet.
2. Pour a drizzle of the olive oil over the vegetable and put the salt and pepper on it as you like. Then add on your

chicken thighs that are seasoned by salt, olive oil, and pepper.

3. Roast in the oven for 15-20 minutes until the skin is brown, and the carrots are tender. You can serve this with a nice salad or steamed vegetables.

Easy Tomato Soup

This recipe takes preparation time of 5 minutes, cooking time of 40 minutes, and creates 6 servings.

A serving contains:
- 3 grams Protein
- 1 grams Carbohydrates
- 8 grams Total fat

What to Use

- Basil (2 tablespoons)
- Heavy cream (0.25 c, low fat if you can find it or the vegan option)
- Salt and Pepper (to taste)
- Chicken bone broth (you can choose whichever broth you want) (2 c)
- Garlic cloves (4 minced)
- Olive oil (2 tablespoons)
- Roma tomatoes (10 medium ones cut into 1" cubes)

What to Do

1. Start your oven to 400 degrees before you start the recipe. Put grease on a baking sheet lightly. Rinse the tomatoes and then chop them into cubes. Then mix the

tomato chunks with minced garlic and extra-virgin olive oil.

2. Roast the tomatoes for about 20-30 minutes in the oven. You can turn them about halfway through so both sides are roasted nicely.

3. When they are roasted, take them out of the oven and cool

4. Then puree the roasted tomatoes in a blender until they are a nice and smooth liquid soup texture.

5. Then put your blended tomato puree into a pot, mix in the broth, plus your seasonings to taste. Cook slowly for a total of 15 minutes.

6. Add in your fresh basil and then the cream. You can serve with toasted bread or a salad.

Grilled Cabbage Steaks

This recipe takes preparation time of 10 minutes, cooking time of 40 minutes, and makes 8 servings.

One single serving contains:

- 4 grams Protein
- 8 g Carbohydrates
- 2 g Fiber
- 3 g Sugar
- 15 grams Total fat

What to Use

- Black Pepper (according to your taste)
- Salt (according to your taste)
- Fresh Juice of a lemon (two tbsp)
- Cooking Oil (Extra-virgin) (0.25 c)
- Garlic (minced) (8 cloves)
- Head of Cabbage
- Bacon (8 slices)

What to Do

- Marinade the Cabbage Steak.

- Fry the bacon and let the bacon fat cool. While the bacon is frying, cut the cabbage into 0.75 inch thick slices. Then in a large bag, add the lemon juice, olive oil, salt and pepper.
- When the bacon fat has cooled enough not to melt the plastic, mix all the ingredients together. Then add the sliced cabbage steaks to the marinade bag and marinate for about 30 minutes. You can switch the position after about 30 minutes so the cabbage can be marinated thoroughly.
- Preheat the grill over medium heat and cook on each side until the edges are crispy and tender or soft.

Cauliflower Nachos with Turkey Meat

This recipe takes preparation time of 15 minutes, cooking time of 25 minutes, and creates 4 portions.

A serving contains:

- 27 g Protein
- 29 g Fat Total
- 14 g Carbohydrates
- 6 g Fiber
- 5 g Sugar

What to Use

- Fresh Cilantro (2 tbsp)
- Avocado (0.5 medium avocado)
- Red onion (sliced 0.3 cup)
- Tomatoes (diced 0.75 cup)
- Cheddar cheese (1 cup shredded)
- Turkey sausage (1 pound)
- Taco seasoning (1 tsp)
- Avocado oil (0.25 cup)
- Cauliflower (1 large head)
- Salsa (optional)
- Guacamole (optional)

1. Start your oven up to 425 degrees. Put grease on your baking sheet and oil it well. Cut the cauliflower into florets and slice them as thinly as possible to make chips. Toss the cauliflower chips with the taco seasoning and avocado oil.

2. Roast them for about 20 minutes on the sheet as a single layer until browned and crispy on the edges.

3. While the cauliflower is roasting, go ahead and cook the turkey sausage for about 10-12 minutes until you do not see any pink.

4. When the cauliflower is finished roasting, flip them over and place the cooked meat over the top of it.

5. Add cheese, red onion, and tomatoes. Then let it in the heat till the cheese melts nicely.

6. You can garnish it with cilantro and avocado. You can add your favorite salsa and guacamole mix or chop a few tomatoes and avocado to make a tomato and avocado salad.

Grilled Salmon and Grapefruit Salad with Olive Oil

This recipe takes preparation time of 15 minutes, cooking time of 10 minutes and creates 4 portions.

A serving contains:

- 21.2 grams Protein
- 2.5 grams Fiber
- 2.1 g Saturated Fat
- 35.8 grams Carbohydrates
- 493 milligrams Sodium
- 2.1 g Polysaturated Fat
- 5.3 grams MSG
- 10 g Total fat

What to Use

- Grapefruit sections (1 24 oz jar)
- Mixed baby salad greens (8 cups)
- Cooking spray
- Large onion (1 cut into 0.5 inch thick slices)
- Ground black pepper (0.25 tsp)
- Salt (.05 tsp)
- Extra-virgin olive oil

1. Get your grill ready. Spread it liberally with cooking spray so the food will not stick to it.
2. Season your salmon, coat with cooking oil or spray and onion slices. Place the onions and fish on the grill rack coated with cooking spray.
3. Then grill until the onion is tender and the fish is flaky.
4. Place two cups of salad greens on four serving plates. Then put the onions into chunks, grapefruit sections, fish, and onion.
5. Then drizzle with extra-virgin olive oil.

Black-Eyed Pea Salad

This recipe takes 15 minutes to prepare, and it makes 4 servings.

A serving contains:

- 6 grams Protein
- 2 grams Sugar
- 4 grams Fiber
- 15 grams Carbohydrates
- 334 milligrams Sodium
- 1.5 grams MSG
- 1 gram Polysaturated Fat
- 3.3 grams Total fat

What to Use

- Baby Arugula (2 c)
- Black-eyed peas (1 15 oz unsalted cans)
- Salt and Pepper (to taste)
- Low-fat or vegan mayo (2.5 tbsp)
- Grape tomatoes (1 cup)

What to Do

1. Before you begin, rinse and drain the black-eyed peas. Combine all the ingredients together. Toss to make sure that it is coated well.
2. Divide among four plates. You can also serve with toasted bread or a few steamed vegetables on the side.

Halibut and Lemon Pesto

This recipe takes preparation time of 3 minutes, cooking time of 8 minutes, and creates portions.

A serving contains:

- 38.7 grams Protein
- 0.5 grams Fiber
- 1.4 grams Carbohydrates
- 363 milligrams Sodium
- 6.3 grams MSG
- 2.3 grams Polysaturated Fat
- 2.6 grams Saturated Fat
- 13 grams Total fat

What to Use

- Juice of a lemon (single tbsp)
- Grated lemon rind (tbsp 1)
- Cloves of garlic (2 peeled)
- Extra-virgin olive oil (2 tbsp)
- Fresh cheese (0.25 c)
- Basil leaves (0.66 c)
- Salt and Pepper (to taste)
- Cooking spray
- Halibut or any firm white fish (4, 6 oz filets)

1. Get your grill ready.
2. Use salt and pepper to season the fish. Put cooking spray or cooking oil on the grill.
3. Grill every side until the fish gets flaky.
4. As the fish grills, make the pesto.
5. Combine a pinch of salt, basil, pepper, garlic cloves, lemon rind, and lemon juice to make the pesto. And blend it all together until it is minced.
6. When it is ready to serve, add a fresh squeeze of lemon juice over the top.

Tomato Granita with an Heirloom Tomato Salad

This recipe takes a preparation time of 15 minutes and makes 6 servings.

A serving contains:

- 1.6 grams Protein
- grams Sugar
- 2.1 grams Fiber
- 0.5 g Polysaturated Fat
- 8.9 grams Carbohydrates
- 0.3 g Saturated Fat
- 174 milligrams Sodium

What to Use

Tomato Salad
- Basil (1 tbsp thinly sliced)
- Salt (according to your taste)
- Black pepper (according to your taste)
- Heirloom tomatoes (2 pounds, which is about 4)

Granita
- Heirloom tomatoes (8 oz seeded and peeled)
- Salt (0.25)
- Olive oil (tsp 2)

- Red wine vinegar (tbsp 1)
- Basil (Fresh) (optional)
- Fresh rosemary (optional)
- Fresh parsley (optional)

What to Do

1. To make the salad, slice the tomatoes and put it on a plate. Then sprinkle your black pepper and salt over the tomatoes. You can also add a few sprigs of fresh parsley, fresh rosemary, or fresh basil.
2. To make the granita, put the extra-virgin olive oil, a 0.25 teaspoon of salad and the peeled, seeded tomato, and vinegar in a powerful blender. Blend all the ingredients until they are smooth. Then freeze it until it is firm.
3. Stir it two times, minimum, in the first 2 hours. Then move the mixture from the fixture and use a fork to fluff it up.
4. You can sprinkle it over the top of your heirloom tomato salad.

Dinner

Lentil Mushroom Tacos

These instructions require 5 minutes of preparation time, cooking time of 20 minutes and create 6 servings.

A serving contains:

- 14 grams Protein
- 3 grams Sugar
- 10 grams Fiber
- 40 grams Carbohydrates
- 936 milligrams Potassium
- 450 milligrams Sodium
- 1 gram Total fat

What to Use

- Water (0.5 cups)
- Cayenne Pepper (teaspoon of 0.5)
- Cumin (teaspoon of 0.5)
- Smoke paprika (0.5 teaspoon)
- Garlic powder (teaspoon of 0.5)
- Salt (according to your taste)
- Chili powder (tablespoon =1)
- Baby Bella mushrooms (a 16 oz package)

- Lentils (2 cups)
- Toasted bread (optional)
- Steamed vegetables (optional)
- Lettuce wraps for the tortilla (optional)
- Low-fat or non-dairy cheese (optional)

What to Do

1. Before you begin, have your lentils already prepared.
2. Then wash the mushrooms and chop them well. Then sauté the mushrooms in a skillet until they are soft. You do not have to add any oil as mushrooms give out a lot of moisture. If you feel the mushrooms are sticking, you can add a little water.
3. Then add the cooked lentils, water, and seasonings, mixing them well.
4. Simmer the mixture until everything is heated through.
5. You can serve in a lettuce tortilla for a healthier option. You can also serve with a side of mixed vegetables or sprinkle dairy or low-fat cheese across the top when it finished cooking.

Cucumber Chickpea Salad

These instructions require a preparation time of 10 minutes and create 4 servings.

A serving contains:

- 13 grams Protein
- 6 grams Sugar
- 9 grams Fiber
- 30 grams Carbohydrates
- 272 milligrams Potassium
- 608 milligrams Sodium
- 9 grams MSG
- 11 grams Polysaturated Fat
- 3 grams Saturated Fat
- 25 grams Total fat

What to Use

- Tahini Dressing
- Water (0.25 c to thin)
- Salt (0.23 teaspoon)
- Garlic clove (1 that's minced)
- Lemon zest (1 lemon)
- Juice (1/2 small lemon)

- Balsamic Vinegar (3 tablespoons)
- Tahini (cup = 0.25)

Salad
- Parsley (Chopped and fresh 0.25 cup)
- Red onion (cup =0.25, diced)
- Chickpeas (a 15 oz can, rinsed and drained)
- Cherry tomatoes (1 pint, halved)
- English cucumber (1, chopped)

What to Do

1. Mix all the salad ingredients very well in one bowl.
2. Mix the dressing ingredients, except water, in a separate bowl.
3. Add a tablespoon of water to the dressing until it is as thin or thick as you would like. If you want to thicken it up, add more tahini to the mix.
4. Then add the dressing and stir everything again.
5. Eat or keep it in the refrigerator until it is ready to be eaten. You can serve on toasted bread of your choice or with crackers. You can also dip vegetables into it and enjoy it as a snack.

Raw Corn Radish Salad

The instructions take a preparation time of 10 minutes and create 6 portions.

A serving contains:

- 3 grams Protein
- 4 grams Sugar
- 25 grams Carbohydrates
- 326 milligrams Potassium
- 13 milligrams Sodium

What to Use

- Salt and pepper (to taste)
- Cumin (0.5 teaspoon)
- Smoked paprika (1.5 teaspoon)
- Lime Juice (use 1 or 2)
- Cilantro (0.25 cup)
- Radishes (1 cup, thinly cut)
- Fresh corn kernels (about 4 cups)

1. Wash and chop your radishes and corn. You can cut the kernels off the cob.
2. Then stir everything in a container.
3. Mix them well, taste and adjust your seasonings as needed.
4. You can serve this by itself or even add a few tortilla chips to the side.

Black Bean Salsa Burgers with Potato Circles

This recipe has a preparation time of 5 minutes, a cooking time of 8 minutes and creates 4 portions.

A serving contains:

- 14 grams Protein
- 5 grams Sugar
- 9 grams Fiber
- 74 grams Carbohydrates
- 669 milligrams Potassium
- 318 milligrams Sodium
- 3 grams MSG
- 1 gram Polysaturated Fat
- 1 gram Saturated Fat
- 6 grams Total fat

What to Use

For the Potato Circles
- Paprika (0.4 of teaspoon)
- Oregano (Dried) (0.75 of teaspoon)
- Parsley (Dried) (0.75 of teaspoon)
- Garlic Powder (0.5 teaspoon)
- Baking Potatoes (2 large ones sliced thinly)

For the Burgers

- Extra-virgin olive Oil (1 tablespoon)
- Your favorite salsa (0.25 cup and 2 tablespoons)
- Brown Rice Flour (0.5 of a cup)
- Old Fashion Oats (0.5 of a cup)
- Black beans (a 15 oz cup)
- Lettuce wraps (optional)

What to Do

For the Potato Circles

1. Start your oven to 450 degrees.
2. Mix the potatoes up with the spices, and put them on a baking sheet that has aluminum foil. You can also choose to spray the baking sheet liberally with extra virgin olive instead.
3. Roast them for about 20-30 minutes, tossing them halfway through.

For the Burgers

1. Mash the black beans and all the ingredients except the extra-virgin olive oil into one bowl. If the mixture seems too wet, you can mix in more flour. If your mixture seems too dry, add 1 tablespoon of salsa, one tablespoon at a time.

2. Separate the mixture into four equal sections and flatten them into patties.

3. Refrigerate them for 20 minutes.

4. Then put oil into a skillet and fry each patty until crispy.

5. Eat using your favorite toppings, including your favorite bun. For a healthier option, you can eat the patties in a lettuce wrap. You can also choose to add a low-fat or non-dairy cheese option to the burger as your 'cheese.'

Green Vegetable Juice with Apple

This recipe takes 5 minutes to prepare and it makes 1 serving.

A serving contains:

- 1 gram Protein
- 8 grams Sugar
- 3 grams Fiber
- 13 grams Carbohydrates
- 191 milligrams Potassium
- 10 milligrams Sodium

What to Use

- A sweet Apple (1 peeled and cored)
- Fresh parsley (a large handful)
- Kale leaf (1 large one)
- Romaine leaves (3)
- Cucumber (half of a medium sized one)
- Raspberries, cherries or blueberries (optional)
- Chia seeds or hemp seeds (optional)
- Protein powder (optional)

1. Wash all of your ingredients well and juice them all until smooth.
2. Drink as soon as you finish.
3. You can modify this by adding green or white tea, apple juice, aloe vera juice, low-fat yogurt, Greek yogurt or water to thin it out.
4. You can also garnish with nuts or seeds or extra fruit. For an extra dose of protein, add a scoop of your favorite protein powder to the mix.

Soba Noodle Stirfry

This recipe takes a preparation time of 10 minutes, cooking time of 5 minutes, and makes 3 servings.

One serving contains:

- 10 g Protein
- 12 g Sugar
- 1001 mg Sodium
- 29 g Carbohydrates
- 4 g Fiber
- 5 grams MSG
- 4 grams Polysaturated Fat
- 2 grams Saturated Fat
- 330 mg Potassium
- 12 grams Total fat

What to Use

- Chopped Peanuts (garnish)
- Ginger (0.25 of a teaspoon)
- Powdered Garlic (0.5 of a teaspoon)
- Pure Maple Syrup (a tablespoon)
- Water (two tablespoons)
- Soy Sauce or Amino Acids (2 tablespoons)
- Rice vinegar (3 tablespoons)

- Natural Peanut Butter (3 tablespoons)
- Onions (Green) (3 thinly sliced)
- Bell Pepper (Red) (Sliced in strips)
- Pepper flakes (optional)
- Hot sauce (optional)

  Soba Noodles (1 9 oz package)

What to Do

1. Boil a pot of water for the noodles. Once the water starts to boil, whisk the amino acids, water, peanut butter, rice vinegar, garlic powder, and ginger in a small bowl and put to the side.
2. Then chop your vegetables. Once the water is boiling, cook the noodles. They do not take long. Please do not overcook or the noodles will be soggy.
3. In a large pan, place 2-3 tablespoons of water and sauté your veggies. After cooking, drain and combine with sautéed vegetables.
4. Then put the sauce over them both and garnish with peanuts. You can also drizzle your favorite hot sauce or a few pepper flakes with a dose of extra heat.

Arugula and Grapefruit Salad

This recipe takes a preparation time of 10 minutes. It makes 2 servings.

A serving contains:

- 4 g Protein
- 4 g Fiber
- 21 g Carbohydrates
- 2 g Sugar
- 580 milligrams Potassium
- 16 milligrams Sodium
- 24 grams MSG
- 4 grams Polysaturated Fat
- 4 grams Saturated Fat
- 30 grams Total fat

What to Use

- Salt and pepper (according to your taste)
- Cooking Oil (Extra-virgin olive oil) (tablespoons = 3 or 4)
- Lemon juice of 1 lemon
- Avocado (0.5 scooped out and mashed)
- Sliced raw almonds (0.125 cups)
- Grapefruit (1 segmented)
- Arugula (4 cups)

1. Wash your arugula and peel your grapefruit. You can even consider putting the arugula in a salad spinner to get it drier.
2. Toss the grapefruit sections, almonds, and arugula together in a bowl.
3. Mix your water, salt, lemon juice, pepper, and avocado together.
4. Drizzle a bit of the mixture over the salad before serving.
5. You can serve with raw cut vegetables like julienned zucchini slices or carrots.

Roasted Drumsticks and Carrots

This recipe takes a preparation time of 20 minutes, cooking time of 40 minutes and makes 6 servings.

A serving contains:

- 25 grams Protein
- 3 grams Sugar
- 7 grams Carbohydrates
- 19 grams Total fat

What to Use

- Salt and Pepper (to taste)
- Cherry Tomatoes (3 c and halved)
- Drumsticks (6)
- Smoked paprika (1 tsp)
- Red onion (cut into 8 wedges)
- Garlic cloves (3 minced)

What to Do

1. Start your oven at 400 degrees. Put grease on your baking pan. Arrange the garlic, onion, and tomatoes in a single layer and put one tablespoon of oil to prevent sticking.

2. Put the spices on the drumstick and position the seasoned chicken sticks on top of the vegetables.

3. Roast the vegetables and chicken for about 30 to 40 minutes until the chicken is fully cooked. You can turn halfway through to prevent sticking.

Chicken and White Bean Soup

These instructions require 2 minutes or preparation time, a preparation time of 13 minutes to cook, and makes 6 servings.

A serving contains:

- 18 grams Protein
- 1.8 grams Fiber
- 8.5 grams Carbohydrates
- 623 milligrams Sodium
- 0.5 g of Saturated Fat
- 3 grams Fat in Total recipe
- 0.6 grams MSG
- 0.5 g of Polysaturated Fat

What to Use

- Green salsa (0.5 c)
- White Beans of your choice (1 16 oz)
- Chicken broth (2 14 oz cans)
- Extra-virgin olive oil
- Chicken breasts (2 cups shredded and cooked)
- Siracha (optional)
- Low-fat or non-dairy cheese (optional)

1. Sauté the chicken in a skillet or pot coated with extra-virgin olive oil. Sauté for about 2 minutes until the chicken is a little bit brown.

2. Add the broth to the skillet and then make sure all the brown bits are scraped so they can mix to the broth.

3. Mash the beans in a different bowl until a few of the whole beans are left.

4. Then you can add the salsa and beans to the broth in the pan or skillet, and stir it well. Bring to the point that it boils. Cook slowly until thick.

5. Once the soup is ready, you can serve with bread, salad or vegetables.

   To take the recipe to another level, you can sprinkle a little low-fat or non-dairy cheese over the top.

6. You can also drizzle a spicy sauce like siracha over the top for an extra kick of heat, too.

Lamb Chops In Orange-Vinegar Sauce

These instructions require a cooking time of 15 minutes, a cooking time of 10 minutes, and create 8 portions.

A serving contains:

- 12.1 grams of Total Fat
- 25 grams Protein
- 2 grams Carbohydrates
- 5.4 grams Monosaturated fat
- 582 milligrams Sodium
- 0.6 grams of Polysaturated fat
- 2 grams Sugar
- 4.6 grams of Saturated fat

What to Use

- Olive oil (tsp 4)
- Grated orange rind (tsp 2)
- Orange juice (tbsp 1)
- Cooking spray
- Lamb rib chops (8 (4-oz) fat trimmed)
- Salt (according to your taste)
- Black pepper (according to your taste)
- Balsamic vinegar (3 tbsp)

1. Before you begin, wash your lamb well. Make sure that your work space has your raw meat separate from your vegetables and other food to prevent cross-contamination.

2. Combine a tablespoon of orange juice, olive oil, and orange rinds in one plastic bag large enough for the marinade. Marinate the lamb well for at least 10 minutes at room temperature.

3. Remove and then season well with seasoning.

4. Warm up the grill and coat it with a liberal amount of cooking spray. Then cook the lamb chops on both sides for about 2 minutes until it is done to your preference.

5. Then take the lamb chops off and place the balsamic vinegar in a small skillet. Cook until the balsamic vinegar is syrupy (maybe about 3 minutes). Put a tablespoon of extra-virgin olive oil. Then drizzle the vinegar and the mixture over the lamb chops.

6. This would be awesome with a corn on the cob or even a small leafy salad, spread with the same vinaigrette sauce.

Pineapple Rice with Grilled Steak

This recipe requires 15 minutes of preparation time, cooking time of 20 minutes and creates 4 portions.

A serving contains:

- 345 milligrams Sodium
- 31 g of Protein
- 52 milligrams Calcium
- 44 g of Carbohydrates
- 6 grams Sugar
- 2.8 grams Saturated fat
- 3 grams Monosaturated fat
- 0.4 grams Polysaturated fat
- 4 grams of Fiber
- 10.3 grams Fat

What to Use

- Black pepper (0.5 tsp)
- Salt (0.9 tsp)
- Precooked Brown Rice (8.8-oz)
- Soy sauce (light sodium) (0.25 c)
- Beef tenderloin fillets (4 (4-oz))
- Cooking spray
- Pineapple slices (1 (8-oz) can, drained)

- Green onions (6 pieces)

What to Do

- Make sure your meat is well washed and the fat is trimmed before you begin the recipe.
- In a large plastic bag, mix together the low-salt, soy sauce, pepper, and beef. Let the beef marinate and stay at a room temperature for about 7 minutes. Turn the bag every now and then so the marinade mixes with the beef well. The more the marinade gets in the meat, the more it will be flavorful.
- While the steak marinates, heat the grilling pan sprayed with cooking oil. Put the green onions and pineapples in the grill and cook it until they are well-charred. Once they are cool, cut the onions and pineapples into bite-sized pieces.
- Cook the pre-cooked rice according to the directions. Then add the pineapples and the green onions to the rice. Once the rice is done, then cook the beef in the grill pan until it is done. You can grill it for 3 minutes on each side until it is done or cooked to how you like it. When it is finished cooking, you can serve the beef with the pineapple rice.

Zucchini and Peas Tortellini Salad

These instructions require a preparation time of 10 minutes, cooking time of 45 minutes, and create 4 portions.

One serving contains:

- 14 grams Total Fat
- 7 g of Fiber
- 3.2 grams of fat that is saturated
- 6.8 grams Monosaturated fat
- 1.6 grams of fat that is polysaturated
- 561 milligrams Sodium
- 34 g of Carbohydrates
- 12 g of Protein
- 5 grams Sugar

What to Use

- Salt (0.5 tsp)
- Black pepper (0.5 tsp)
- 3-cheese tortellini (9 ounce package)
- Zucchini (2 medium ones zoodles)
- Frozen peas (0.6 c)
- Grated lemon rind (tsp 1)
- Olive oil (tbsp 2)
- Minced cloves of garlic (2 total)

- Lemon juice (1 tbsp)
- Fresh basil (optional)

What to Do

1. Prepare the tortellini. Add peas towards the end of the tortellini when its almost ready. When the tortellini is ready, pour the water off, and let it cool. Cut the zucchini into small thin ribbons.
2. Cook the garlic in oil then add the zucchini noodle and cook until the zucchini is soft.
3. Mix the rind of the lemon, juice of the lemon, pepper, and salt with the olive oil. Drizzle it over tortellini mixture. Put the tortellini in the mixture and top with basil.
4. This would be great served with a fruit cocktail or medley.

Turkey Sausage in Gnocchi Soup

This recipe has a preparation time of 5 minutes, a cooking time of 12 minutes and creates 7 servings.

A serving contains:

- 4 grams Fat
- 1.7 grams Saturated fat
- 10.5 grams Protein
- 25.1 grams Carbohydrates
- 0.5 grams Fiber
- 809 milligrams Sodium

What to Use

- Turkey Italian sausage (4.5 oz)
- Water (2 c)
- Gnocchi (16-oz pack)
- Beef broth (14-oz can, low-fat and low-sodium)
- Italian-style stewed tomatoes (14.5-oz can, chopped)
- Low-fat parmesan cheese (0.5 c)

1. Cook the sausage until it begins to crumble. You can substitution a vegan meat or meatless patty to make it healthier.

2. Then add 2 cups water to the pan then the broth, tomatoes, and gnocchi. Boil everything together, and then cook it slow when it starts boiling or until the gnocchi comes to the top of the pot.

3. Divide the soup, and then spread the cheese over the top of the bowls. You can also substitute a vegan cheese or omit it altogether for a healthier option.

Shrimp Sausage

This recipe takes a preparation time of 6 minutes, a cooking time of 9 minutes, and creates 4 servings.

A serving contains:

- 1 gram of Saturated fat
- .1 grams of Monosaturated fat
- .3 grams of Polysaturated fat
- 3 grams Fat
- 19 g of Protein
- 7.6 g of Carbohydrates
- .6 grams of Fiber
- 701 milligrams Sodium
- 48 milligrams Calcium

What to Use

- Cooking spray
- Old Bay seasoning (1 tsp)
- Water (0.25 c)
- Black pepper (0.25 tsp)
- Medium shrimp (0.75 pounds, peeled and deveined)
- Tri-color bell pepper (1 c pre-chopped)
- Smoked turkey sausage, (6.5-oz cut into slices)
- Mined cloves of garlic (2)

1. Heat up a skillet sprayed with cooking oil or cooking spray. Add the shrimp and seasoning. Toss while cooking until it is done. Remove the heat and keep it warm.

2. Add more cooking oil or cooking spray. Then put the bell pepper, turkey sausage, shrimp mixture, and garlic. Then add the water.

3. Make sure to stir everything so it does not burn. Make sure all the brown on the bottom is scraped up to spread the extra flavor around the dish.

4. You can serve this with noodles that have been thinly sliced or cut into ribbons with a zoodler. To make it healthier, you can substitute meatless meat for the sausage.

Portobello Pizza

The instructions require 10 minutes of preparation time, a cooking time of 20 minutes, and it makes 4 servings.

A serving contains:

- 6 grams Fat
- 7 grams Protein
- 5 grams Carbohydrates
- 4 grams Net Carbs
- 1 gram Fiber
- 3 grams Sugar

What to Use

- Olive oil spray
- Pepperoni or turkey or meatless sausage (16 slices)
- Portobello mushrooms (4 large ones)
- Marinara sauce (0.5 c)
- Low-fat mozzarella shredded cheese (0.5 c)

What to Do

1. Start your stove to 375 degrees. Put aluminum foil on a baking sheet. Coat it well with a layer of olive oil spray.
2. Using a spoon, scrape out the dark gills from the mushrooms and throw the gills away.

3. Put the mushrooms with their stems facing up, and top each one with 2 tbsp of marinara sauce. Also sprinkle each with 2 tbsp low-fat mozzarella, and 4 slices of the meat you want.

4. Bake them for 20 - 25 minutes or the cheese is bubbling or the mushrooms are soft. You can also serve with a salad.

Sweet Potato, Leek and Ham Soup

This recipe takes a preparation time of 6 minutes, cooking time of 28 minutes, and it creates 4 portions.

A serving contains:

- .1 gram of Polysaturated Fat
- .2 g of Saturated Fat
- .2 g of Monosaturated Fat
- 1 gram Fat
- 15.5 grams Protein
- 29.2 grams Carbohydrates
- 3.6 grams Fiber
- 625 milligrams Sodium

What to Use

- Olive oil-flavored cooking spray
- Leek (1 .5 c thinly sliced)
- Green onions (thinly sliced)
- Water (2 c)
- Pepper (0.25 tsp)
- Chicken broth (1 c fat-free, less-sodium)
- Evaporated fat-free milk (5 oz can)
- Sweet potato (3 c refrigerated, cubed and peeled)
- Cooked ham (1 c diced)

What to Do

1. Spray a pot or Dutch oven with a cooking spray and brown the ham. When it is brown to your liking, set it to the side.

2. Add the leeks to the pan and coat with cooking spray. Cook them until they are tender. To prevent burning, you can add some water.

3. Then add the sweet potatoes, onions, chicken broth, and evaporated fat-free milk. Scrape the loosened brown bits. Cook slowly until the sweet potatoes are tender.

4. Then blend half of the soup and pour the blended half into a separate container. Then do the same thing with the remaining soup. Return both blended halves back to the Dutch oven.

5. Put in rest of the ham. Serve the soups. You can garnish with salad, onions and ham. A slice or a few slices of nice thick toasty bread would be a welcome addition, too.

Chili with Beef, Corn and Black Beans

This recipe takes a preparation time of 3 minutes, a cooking time of 30 minutes, and it makes 6 servings.

A serving contains:

- 1 gram Saturated Fat
- 20 g Protein
- 1 gram Monosaturated Fat
- 3 g of Fiber
- 0.3 grams Polysaturated Fat
- 3 grams Fat
- 825 mg Sodium
- 20 grams Carbohydrates

What to Use

- Ground round (1 pound)
- Sliced green onions
- Salt-free chili powder (2 tsp)
- Corn and Black beans (1 frozen package, seasoned if possible)
- Beef broth (1 can fat-free and less sodium)
- Seasoned tomato sauce (1 can)

1. Mix the beef and chili powder in a frying skillet. Cook the beef until it is brown and crumbly. Drain the grease away from the meat and return the meat and chili powder mixture back into your pan.

2. Add the broth, tomato sauce, and corn mixture. Bring to a boil, then turn it down and cook it slowly. For the last 5 minutes, uncover it and let it simmer.

3. Scoop the warm chili into bowls carefully. Add the sliced green onions to the top as a garnish. You can serve with toasted sprouted bread. You can also serve with a leafy salad. For maximum health, you can put the mixture into leaf wraps and eat it like a taco meat substitution.

Smothered Pepper Steak

This recipe takes a preparation time of 4 minutes to prepare, a cooking time of 25 minutes, and creates 4 servings.

A serving contains:

- 8 grams of Fat
- 18 g Carbohydrates
- 2 grams Saturated Fat
- 2 g of Fiber
- 2 grams Monosaturated Fat
- 0.5 grams Polysaturated Fat
- 25 g of Protein
- 785 milligrams Sodium

What to Use

- Low-sodium soy sauce (1 tbsp)
- Sirloin patties (4 ground ones)
- Cooking spray
- Salt (according to your taste)
- All-purpose flour (tbsp 3)
- Black pepper (according to your taste)
- Frozen bell pepper stir-fry (1 package)
- Diced tomatoes (a can, undrained, with olive oil, basil and balsamic vinegar)

1. Place the flour in a shallow dish. Then season the sirloin patties, and then dredge the sirloin patties in flour.

2. Spray your frying skillet with cooking oil or cooking spray and heat it up. Fry each side until brown on each side.

3. Add the stir-fry frozen mixture, soy sauce, and canned tomatoes to the patties in the frying pan and let it boil.

4. Once boiling, turn the heat down and cook it slower for 15 minutes or until meat is done and gravy is thickened.

5. You can serve this with a salad or a steamed vegetable medley. If you want a meatless option, you can use eggplant in place of the sirloin patties and get the same crispy, meaty effect.

Salmon, Avocado, and Sweet Kale Salad with a Lemon Vinaigrette

This recipe takes 5 minutes to prepare, and it makes 6 servings.

A serving contains:

- 14 grams Fat
- 7 grams Protein
- 10 grams Total Carbs
- 7 grams Net Carbs
- 3 grams Fiber
- 4 grams Sugar

What to Use

Salmon, Avocado, and Sweet Kale Salad
- Sweet Kale Salad Mix (1 12-ounce bag)
- Blueberries (1 c)
- Smoked salmon (4-ounce cut into bite-size pieces)
- Shelled Pistachios (0.33 c)
- Avocado (0.5 of a medium avocado, cut in cubes)

Lemon Vinaigrette Dressing
- Mayonnaise or vegan mayo (0.25 of a c)
- Oil (Olive) (tbsp =1)

- Juice of a lemon (tbsp=1)
- Powdered garlic (0.25 of tsp)
- Sweetener (2 tbsp)
- Poppy seeds (1 tsp)

What to Do

- Smoke your salmon. Then combine the salad mix, salmon, and blueberries. Then combine the blueberries and smoked salmon.
- Mix all the dressing ingredients together. You can whisk it together. Then toss the dressing with the salad.
- Crush the pistachios. Then add the pistachios and cubed avocado to the salad, and then toss the salad again.
- You can also add a few pepper flakes to make it have an extra quick.

Broccoli Cranberry Salad with Bacon Walnuts

These instructions require a preparation time of 10 minutes and create 10 servings.

A serving contains:

- 11 grams Fat
- 4 grams Protein
- 5 grams Total Carbohydrates
- 1.5 grams Fiber
- 1.5 grams Sugar

What to Use

Broccoli Cranberry Salad
- Sugar-free dried cranberries (0.5 c)
- Walnuts (0.5 c, chopped)
- Bacon bits (0.5 c)
- Broccoli (1 bunch, chopped into small florets)
- Red onion (0.25 c sliced)

Creamy Lemon Poppy Seed Dressing
- Garlic powder (0.5 tsp)
- Poppy seeds (0.5 tsp)
- Salt (to taste)
- Pepper (to taste)

- Mayonnaise or vegan mayo (0.5 c)
- Oil Olive (tbsp 1)
- Zest Orange (tsp 1)
- Juice of a lemon (1 tbsp)
- Your choice of sweetener (1.5 tbsp)

What to Do

1. Combine all the salad together: chopped broccoli, red onion, bacon bits, cranberries, and walnuts.
2. Using a completely separate bowl, whisk the mayonnaise, olive oil, lemon juice, garlic powder, orange zest, sweetener, and poppy seeds. Adjust the sweetener of your choice to taste. Then season it with pepper and salt.
3. Finally, pour the lemon poppy seed dressing into the vegetable mixture. Refrigerate for an hour or more for better flavor.
4. For a meatless option, go for meat-free bacon bits or forget the bacon altogether. If you do not like walnuts, you can skip them or substitute it with your favorite walnut. This would pair well with a smoothie, too.

Spinach, Hummus and Bell Pepper Wraps

These instructions require a preparation time of 10 minutes and create 2 servings.

A serving contains:

- 12.1 g of Fat
- 15 g of Protein
- 13 g of Fiber
- 34 g of Carbohydrates
- 793 mg Sodium
- 7 g of Sugar
- 2.9 g of Saturated Fat
- 5.6 g of Monosaturated Fat
- 3 grams Polysaturated Fat

What to Use

- Roasted garlic hummus (0.5 c)
- Red bell pepper (1 small one thinly sliced)
- Tomato-and-basil feta cheese (0.25 c)
- Baby spinach (1 c firmly packed together)
- Whole-grain flatbreads (2)

1. Spread each side of the flatbread with 0.25 cup of hummus, leaving small space of border.
2. Split the bell pepper slices evenly amongst the flatbread.
3. Add spinach and cheese on each one. Then roll up the wraps and stick a toothpick through it to hold it. You can split the rolls in half if you would like.
4. To take the recipe to the next level, you can use lettuce wraps instead of a grain-based wraps.

Desserts and Snacks

No-Bake Peanut Butter Cookies

These instructions require a preparation time of 10 minutes; it makes 12 cookies.

A serving is one cookie, and it contains:

- 3.8 grams Protein
- 16.2 grams Sugar
- 3.9 mg of Sodium
- 2.9 grams Fiber
- 24.5 grams Carbohydrates
- 6.2 g of Total fat
- 1.2 g of Saturated fat

What to Use

- Natural salted peanut butter (0.5 c)
- Pitted Medjool date (0.75 c)
- Rolled oats, gluten-free (1 c)
- Sea salt (a smidget)
- Dark chocolate (optional)
- Agave or honey (optional)

What to Do

1. Add salt and oats to a blender and pulse until it is a flour consistency. You can add the dates and blend for 30 more seconds. Then add peanut butter and blend it all together until it forms.

2. Scoop out to the tablespoon amounts of dough and form into small balls. Put on a parchment lined tray.

3. You can drizzle with dark chocolate that was melted in the microwave for a little extra sweetness. If you do not like chocolate, you can substitute agave or honey instead.

Easy Shortbread

The instructions require a preparation time of 15 minutes, a cooking time of 20 minutes, and create 48 servings.

A serving contains:

- 1 grams Protein
- 5 grams Sugar
- 12 grams Carbohydrates
- 62 milligrams Sodium
- 5 grams Saturated Fat
- 8 grams Total fat

What to Use

- Flour (all-purpose) (4 to 4.5 c)
- Sugar (brown) (1 c)
- Butter (2 c softened)

What to Do

1. Start your oven up to 325 degrees. Combine the butter and brown sugar together. Add in the flour, about 3.75 cups and combine. Knead and work the dough on a floured surface to make dough that is soft.

2. Roll the dough and cut into 1-inch strips. Place them on an ungreased cookie sheet. Make holes with a fork. Bake for at least 20 minutes until the cookies are browned. Cook for up to 25 minutes.

3. This would pair well with a fruit for a healthy snack or dessert. This recipe also freezes well so you can make a huge batch and freeze them to be eaten at a later date.

Butterscotch and Dark Chocolate Haystacks

These instructions require 10 minutes to prepare and make 20 servings.

One serving contains:

- 1 grams Protein
- 15 grams Sugar
- 1 grams Fiber
- 22 grams Carbohydrates
- 84 milligrams Sodium
- 5 grams Saturated Fat
- 9 grams Total fat

What to Use

- Crispy chow mein noodles (4 c)
- Butterscotch chips (1 10-11 ounce package)
- Semisweet dark chocolate chips (2 c)

What to Do

1. Melt the chocolate chips and the butterscotch chips in a large metal bowl over simmering water or in a microwave. Watch it to make sure it doesn't burn.

2. Add wax parchment to a baking sheet. Then drop the rounded tablespoon. Set it by putting it into the refrigerator for 10-15 minutes or until it is set. These are a crowd favorite and very easy to make.

3. You can also substitute the dark chocolate for your favorite chocolate. Another way to modify this dessert is if you add a little bit of cayenne pepper to make it a spicy hot combination.

Veggie Chip Clusters

This recipe takes 15 minutes to prepare, and it makes 36 servings.

A serving contains:

- 1 grams Sugar
- 1 g of Saturated Fat
- 2 grams Carbohydrates
- 19 mg of Sodium
- 3 g of Total fat

What to Use

- Chopped pecans or your favorite nut (0.5 c)
- Veggie chips (2 c, ridged and coarsely crushed)
- White baking chocolate (9 oz)

What to Do

1. In the microwave or in a large metal bowl in simmering water, melt the white chocolate. Then stir in the nuts and veggie chips. Add wax paper onto a baking sheet. Then drop them by the tablespoon full. Refrigerate for 15-20 minutes until set.

2. You can experiment with different types of veggies chips or different types of chocolate to come up with your favorite combination.

Easy Bunny Tails

These instructions require a preparation time of 20 minutes and make 48 servings.

A serving contains:

- 3 grams Sugar
- 3 grams Carbohydrates
- milligrams Potassium
- 1 grams Saturated Fat
- 2 grams Total fat

What to Use

- Sweetened Shredded Coconut (1 c)
- White baking chips (1 c, melted)

What to Do

1. Put wax paper onto a baking sheet.
2. Then drop the melted chocolate onto the waxed paper. You can also use parchment paper. Then sprinkle each ball with the coconut flakes. Let them rest until they are completely dry.

3. This is very easy to make. You can also make it healthier by using any type of chocolate you'd like, like dark chocolate or a vegan or dairy-free chocolate.

Layered Lemon Pie

These instructions require a preparation time of 20 minutes, a setting time of 15 minutes and make 6 servings.

A serving contains:

- 1 g of Fiber
- 61 g of Sugar
- 72 g Carbohydrates
- 13 grams Saturated Fat
- 251 mg Sodium
- 24 grams Total fat
- 6 g of Protein

What to Use

- Graham cracker or your favorite type of nut crust (9 inches)
- Low-fat frozen whipped topping (1 8 oz, thawed)
- Lemon pie filling (1 can, divided into two equal parts)
- Sugar (0.5 c)
- Cream cheese (Low-fat or vegan) (8 oz)

1. Cream the sugar and cream cheese together. Beat in the pie filling, about half. Fold topping that is whipped then spoon into the crust.

2. Put the leftover lemon filling on the top of the cream cheese laver.

3. Let it set for a minimum of 15 minutes by putting it into the refrigerator right up until the serving time.

4. When you are ready to serve, you can serve it with green or white tea.

Creamy Pineapple Pie

These instructions require a preparation time of 10 minutes and make 6 servings.

One serving contains:

- 1 gram of Fiber
- 185 mg Sodium
- 46 g of Sugar
- 54 g Carbohydrates
- 5 g of Protein
- 9 grams Saturated Fat
- 14 grams Total fat

What to Use

- Macadamia nuts (optional, chopped and toasted)
- Additional crushed pineapple (optional)
- Graham cracker crust (1 9-inch one)
- Low-fat, frozen whipped topping (1 8 oz carton)
- Lemon juice (0.25 cup)
- Crushed pineapple (1 8 oz can, drained)
- Sweetened condensed milk (1 14 oz can)

1. If you decided to toast the nuts, bake them for at least 5 minutes, no longer than 10 minutes at 350 degrees or roast in a skillet over low heat, constantly turning them until they are light brown.

2. To make the pie, you combine the sweetened condensed milk, crushed pineapple, and lemon juice and then fold it into the low-fat frozen whipped topping.

3. Then pour it into the graham cracker crust. Refrigerate it until it is ready to be served. You can garnish it with the toasted macadamia nuts and additional crushed pineapples if you would like.

Bakeless Kiwi Cheesecake

These instructions require at least 25 minutes of preparation time, a freeze time of at least 3 hours, and make 6 servings.

A serving contains:

- 24 g of Carbohydrates
- 3 g of Fiber
- 16 g of Sugar
- 2 g of Protein
- 8 g of Total fat

What to Use

For the topping
- Blueberries (optional)
- Raspberries (optional)
- Fresh mint
- SunGold Kiwis (2)
- Green Kiwi (1)

For the cheesecake layer
- Green kiwi (1)
- Mint leaves (1)
- Agave or rice syrup (tbsp 2)

- Lime juice (2 tbsp)
- Milk (Coconut or non-dairy) (0.75 full-fat)
- Cashews (2 c, soaked for at least 4-6 hours or at least overnight)

For the crust
- Dates (1 c)
- Almonds (1 c)

What to Do

1. Pulse almonds until nicely crushed. Then add the dates and blend them again until a sticky mixture forms. Then press it into a 7-inch springform pan, and put in into the freezer.
2. Next, make the cheesecake layer by draining the cashews. Combine the cashews with the coconut milk, lime juice and agave in a blender until it becomes creamy and smooth.
3. Then put about 75% of the cashew mixture evenly onto the base layer and put it back into the freezer.
4. Leave the rest of it in the blender, and add one kiwi, then the fresh mint leaves. Blend it all together up until the mixture is smooth and light green. Put it on top of the already freezing layers, and put it back in the freezer for 2-3 hours.

5. Take it out about 20-30 minutes before it is ready to serve. You can drizzle it with agave or rice syrup and then top it with the fruit.

6. This is a very popular dessert. It also pairs well with a hot drink like a green tea or infused lemon water.

Super Easy Blueberry Ice Cream

This recipe takes 5 minutes to prepare, and it makes 2 servings.

A serving contains:

- 3 mg of Sodium
- 6 g Fiber
- 41 g Carbohydrates
- 485 mg Potassium
- 24 g Sugar
- 2 g Protein
- 0.1 grams monosaturated fat
- 0.4 grams Polysaturated Fat
- 0.2 grams Saturated Fat
- 1 gram Total fat

What to Use

- Frozen blueberries (1.5 c)
- Bananas (2 ripe ones)
- Strawberries, raspberries, blueberries (optional)
- Chia seeds (optional)

1. The night before you make this, slice the bananas and freeze them overnight.
2. Then put them in the blender with the frozen blueberries and blend them together until it is smooth. Be sure to scrape the sides down while it is blending.
3. Then top it off with fresh strawberries, raspberries, blueberries, granola, and coconut chips. To make it even healthier, you can add in chia seeds.

Simple Lemon Bark

These instructions require an hour and 10 minutes of preparation time and make 1.75 pounds of servings.

A serving contains:

- 1 gram Protein
- 14 grams Sugar
- 15 grams Carbohydrates
- 20 milligrams Sodium
- 4 grams Saturated Fat
- 7 grams Total fat

What to Use

- Hard lemon candies (1 c, low-fat option, divided into equal parts)
- White baking chips (2 10-12 ounce packages

What to Do

1. Put foil in a 15 x 10 x 1-inch pan. Then warm the baking chips in a metal bowl over simmering water until it is melted.
2. Be careful and watch it to prevent it from burning. Stir in most of the candy. Leave only a little to put on top.

3. Refrigerate it for about 1 hour until it is set. Then break it into pieces.

4. For a healthier option, you can look for vegan lemon candy.

Sweet Power Balls

These instructions require a preparation time of 45 minutes and it makes 25 servings.

The serving size is 1 ball; it contains:

- 19 milligrams calcium
- 72 milligrams potassium
- 13 milligrams sodium
- .6 milligrams iron
- 1 grams fiber
- 1.4 grams carbohydrates
- .7 grams protein

What to Use

- Shredded unsweetened coconut (.75 c)
- Honey (.5 c)
- Room temperature sunflower butter (.3 c)
- Sesame seeds (.25 c)
- Semisweet chocolate chips (.3 c)
- Diced dried plums (.5 c)
- Puffed rice (1 c)
- Puffed millet (.5 c)

1. Mix the puffed millet and rice together with dried plums, sesame seeds, and chocolate chips.

2. Mix in the honey and sunflower buttons and then cover and refrigerate in the bowl for a total of 30 minutes.

3. Put the shredded coconut in a separate bowl. Then using a tablespoon, scoop the mixture and form it into a 2.5 cm ball. Shape the ball with your hands and roll the balls in the shredded coconut and put in a container.

4. A healthy modification would be to use dark chocolate chips.

Spicy-Sweet Fruit Salad

This recipe takes 10 minutes to make and makes 6 servings.

A serving contains:

- 1.3 grams Protein
- 20.6 grams Sugar
- 3.9 grams Fiber
- 27.4 grams Carbohydrates
- 44 milligrams Sodium
- 0.7 grams Fat

What to Use

- Sea Salt (a pinch)
- Chili Powder (0.25 teaspoon)
- Maple Syrup (1 tablespoon)
- Juiced small lime (2 tablespoons)
- Blueberries (1 cup)
  Sliced strawberries (1 cup)
- Kiwi (4 medium ones)
- Mangos (2 ripe ones)

1. Peel and cut all fruit into cubes and place it in a bowl. Mix the lime juice and maple syrup together. Drizzle the mixture over the fruit in the bowl.
2. Then add sea salt and chili powder. Adjust the seasonings to your liking.
3. This is a personal favorite of mine and a very big hit at different potlucks and family gatherings.

Hummus-Zucchini English Muffin

This recipe makes 1 serving.

A serving contains:

- 1.3 grams Saturated Fat
- 0.5 grams Monosaturated Fat
- 1.8 grams Polysaturated Fat
- 8.7 grams Fat
- 8 grams Protein
- 30 grams Carbohydrates
- 6 grams Fiber
- 361 milligrams Sodium
- 2 grams Sugar

What to Use

- Shaved carrot (2 tbsp)
- Shaved zucchini (2 tbsp)
- Hummus (2 tbsp)
- Whole-grain English muffin, (1 divided in half)
- Roasted salted sunflower seeds (2 tbsp)

What to Do

1. Divide the English muffin in half.

2. Use a zoodler to cut the zucchini and carrot thinly or slice it thinly.
3. Spread hummus on each side of English muffin.
4. Then top with carrot, zucchini, and sunflower seeds.
5. You can substitute pumpkin seeds for sunflower seeds. If you do not want to do hummus, you can do guacamole.

Grilled Chicken and Pineapple Sandwiches

These instructions require a preparation time of 6 minutes, a cooking time of 10 minutes, and it makes 4 servings.

A serving contains:

- 0.9 g of Saturated Fat
- 4 grams Total Fat
- 30.5 g of Carbohydrates
- 1 gram of Monosaturated Fat
- 43.4 g of Protein
- 1.4 g of Polysaturated Fat
- 608 mg of Sodium
- 4.1 g of Fiber

What to Use

- Cooking spray
- Boneless and skinless chicken breasts (4 6-oz halves)
- Salt (0.5 tsp)
- Light mayonnaise
- Black pepper (0.25 tsp)
- Juice of 2 fresh limes
- Pineapple slices (4, 0.5-inch thick)
- Whole wheat hamburger buns (4 toasted or lettuce wraps)

- Basil (4 large leaves)

What to Do

1. Prepare grill and spray a lot of cooking spray liberally.
2. Season the chicken well and grill them. Every now and then, brush the chicken with lime juice.
3. Then grill the slices of pineapple and assemble your sandwich by adding chicken, grilled pineapple slice, and a basil leaf to each sandwich.
4. Spread mayonnaise on bottom halves of buns, if desired.
5. A healthy modification is to add a lettuce bun.

Fresh Orange Sorbet

This recipe takes 15 minutes to prepare and 2 hours and 8 minutes to cook, and it makes 12 servings.

A serving contains:

- 0.4 grams Protein
- 23.1 grams Carbohydrates
- 0.2 grams Fiber
- 1 milligram Sodium
- 5 milligrams Calcium

What to Use

- Oranges (10 medium ones)
- Water (2.5 c)
- Fresh lemon juice (0.33 c)
- Grated orange rind
- Sugar (1 c)
- Mint sprigs (optional)
- Rosemary (optional)

1. Remove the rind and white pit from an orange very carefully. Then cut the orange rind into longwise thin strips.

2. Segment the peeled oranges to half sections, then squeeze the juice until it equals 0.33 cup.

3. Combine the sugar and water to a pan and boil, then add the orange rind strips to pan.

4. Turn the heat down and cook it slowly for 5 minutes. Drain the mixture so no pulp is left. Only save the liquid and discard solids. Cool it.

5. Next, add orange and lemon juice to the sugar liquid, and stir.

6. You can then pour the totality of the liquid mixture into an ice-cream freezer for the tabletop and freeze the orange sorbet as written by the manufacturer.

7. Spoon sorbet into a freezer-safe container; cover and freeze for 1 hour or until firm. You can top it with the grated rind and mint sprigs if desired. You can also add a sprig of rosemary as a garnish.

Mini Zucchini Pizzas

These instructions require a preparation time of 10 minutes, a cooking time of 5 minutes, and make 10 servings.

One serving contains:

- 2 grams Protein
- 1 grams Sugar
- 108 mg of Sodium
- 1 grams Carbohydrates
- 2 g of Total fat
- 1 g of Saturated Fat

What to Use

- Minced basil
- Mini pepperoni or meatless mini pepperoni slices (0.5 c)
- Low-fat mozzarella or vegan cheese (0.75 c)
- Pizza sauce (0.3 c)
- Pepper (0.125 tsp)
- Salt (0.125 tsp)
- Zucchini (1 large one)

What to Do

1. Cut the zucchini diagonally into 0.25-inch slices.

2. Then preheat the broiler. Put the zucchini on a lightly greased baking sheet. Keep it in one single layer.

3. Broil for at least 1 minute up to two minutes on every side until crisp and tender are the zucchini.

4. After you take the zucchini out, use a smidget of salt and pepper on top and add the sauce, pepperoni, and cheese. Broil again for about 1 minute until the cheese is melted. Sprinkle with basil if you would like.

Brownie Batter Bites

This recipe takes 5 minutes to prepare, and it makes 12 servings.

A serving contains:

- 6 grams Protein
- 8 grams Sugar
- 3 grams Fiber
- 12 grams Carbohydrates
- 212 milligrams Potassium
- 8milligrams Sodium
- 4 grams Total fat

What to Use

- Dairy-free chocolate chips (2-4 tbsp)
- Salt (2-4 tbsp)
- Vanilla extract (2 tsp)
- Unflavored pea protein powder (0.25 c)
- Almond butter (0.25 c)

What to Do

1. Put all the ingredients minus the chocolate chips into a bowl and mix it extremely well. You can add a few

teaspoons of water if you ware having trouble mixing it together. Only add it if you need help mixing everything together. We do not want the dough to be too runny since they will be formed into balls.

2. Add in the chocolate chips after you've mixed everything together. Then mix again to make sure everything is properly combined.

3. If you just want to eat it as browning batter, you can eat it that way. If you want to form it as balls, you can roll them into balls and put them on a wax paper lined baking tray or parchment paper. Let it sit for about 15 minutes then put into a container once it finishes setting.

Carrot Cookie Bites

These instructions require a preparation time of 15 minutes, a cooking time of 10 minutes, and create 7 dozen servings.

A serving contains:

- 1 gram Protein
- 3 grams Sugar
- 6 grams Carbohydrates
- 24 milligrams Sodium
- 2 grams Total fat

What to Use

- Pecans (0.5 c chopped)
- Shredded carrots (1 c)
- Quick cooking oatmeal (2 c)
- Ground cloves (tsp 0.25)
- Ground nutmeg (tsp 0.25)
- Soda (Baking) (tsp 0.25)
- Powder (Baking) (tsp 0.25)
- Salt (according to your taste)
- Cinnamon (a tsp)
- All-purpose flour (2 big cups)
- Vanilla extract (a tsp)

- Low-fat Buttermilk (0.5 c)
- Eggs (2 large ones)
- Brown sugar (1 c)
- Shortening (0.66 c)

What to Do

1. Start your oven to 375 degrees.
2. Beat the shortening and brown sugar. Then add in your vanilla, eggs, low-fat buttermilk. Then mix the cinnamon, baking powder, flour, baking soda, nutmeg, cloves, and salt slowly and gradually to the creamed mixture. Then you can stir in the pecans, oats, and carrots.
3. Drop the dough about 2 inches apart by rounded teaspoon onto a baking sheet that is ungreased. Bake for about 6-8 minutes until it is lightly browned. Cool by removing them from the wire racks.

Spinach and Turkey Pinwheels

These instructions require a preparation time of 10 minutes and create 8 portions.

A serving contains:

- 17 grams Protein
- 1 grams Sugar
- 1 grams Fiber
- 31 grams Carbohydrates
- 866 milligrams Sodium
- 6 grams Saturated Fat
- 13 grams Total fat

What to Use

- Sliced Deli Turkey (1 pound)
- Fresh baby spinach (4 cups)
- Tortillas or lettuce wraps (8, 8-inch)
- Low-fat garden vegetable cream cheese (1 8oz carton)

What to Do

1. Spread the cream cheese over the tortillas or lettuce wraps. Then alternate and layer it with turkey and

spinach. Roll it up tightly and stick a toothpick in it. You can refrigerate until it is ready to be served.

Garbanzo Bean Stuffed Baby Peppers

These instructions require a preparation time of 20 minutes and create 32 servings.

A serving contains:

- 1 grams Protein
- 1 grams Sugar
- 1 grams Fiber
- 3 grams Carbohydrates
- 36 milligrams Sodium

What to Use

- Mini Sweet peppers (16, halved lengthwise)
- Salt (0.24 tsp)
- Cider Vinegar (3 tbsp)
- Water (3 tbsp)
- Fresh cilantro leaves (0.25 c)
- Chickpeas (1 can, rinsed and drained)
- Cumin seeds (1 tsp)

1. First, toast the cumin seeds for at least 1 minute, no more than 2 minutes, up to the point that they start to smell nice. Keep stirring them to prevent burning.

2. Once they are toasted, transfer the cumin seeds to a blender and add in the water, vinegar, salt, chickpeas. Then put it on the pulse setting and pulse until everything is well-blended.

3. Then spoon the mixture into pepper halves. Top with extra cilantro. Keep in the fridge until they are ready to be served.

Twice Baked Vegan Sweet Potato Skins

The instructions require a preparation time of 15 minutes, a cooking time of 15 minutes, and create 4 portions.

A serving contains:

- 34 g of Carbohydrates
- 4 g of Protein
- 6 g of Fiber
- 544 mg of Potassium
- 310 mg of Sodium
- 6 g of Sugar

What to Use

- Toppings (Optional)
- Hot sauce
- Chopped cilantro
- Your favorite salsa
- Low-fat or non-dairy cheese sauce
- Avocado
- Sliced green onions
- Sautéed peppers

Potatoes

- Corn (0.25 c, can be thawed frozen corn or fresh)
- Black beans (0.25, drained and rinsed off)
- Hot sauce (2-4 tbsp)
- Diary-free yogurt (0.25 c)
- Salt (smidget)
- Extra-virgin olive oil (drizzle for baking)
- Sweet potatoes (4, 2.5 by 4 inch ones)

What to Do

1. Preheat your oven to 350 degrees Fahrenheit.
2. Wash the potatoes. Then rub them with broth or oil to get the salt to stick.
3. Bake the sweet potatoes in your oven for at least 45 minutes.
4. Once tender, remove them from the oven. Then let them cool for a little bit before slicing them. Then when they are cool, slick them in half.
5. Scoop out the insides. Be sure to leave a small edge on the inside.
6. Once they are scooped out, put the potatoes, inside side down, to crisp the outside of the potatoes.
7. Then mix the potato insides with the yogurt and hot sauce. Add the corn and beans. Mix everything very well together. Take the skins out the oven and put the mixture on the inside of them.

8. Bake it all again for 10-15 minutes.

Then you can top it with whatever toppings you would like.

Conclusion

Thank for making it through to the end of *Anti-Inflammatory Diet for Beginners: The 3 Week Meal Plan to Naturally Restore The Immune System and Heal Inflammation with 84 Proven Easy Recipes*. Let's hope it was informative and able to provide you with all of the tools you need to achieve your goals whatever they may be.

In conclusion, the entire point of the anti-inflammatory diet is to let 'Food be thy medicine' and cure your chronic inflammation. Unfortunately, many diseases that result in chronic inflammation leave doctors confounded. Yet, there is one common denominator and that is what you eat. One of the quickest and cheapest ways to treat your inflammation is through your diet. By focusing on what you put into your body with this diet, it becomes a lifestyle change that can heal and ease your pain.

Remember, the anti-inflammatory lifestyle is not a one-and-done thing. It is a commitment to change in your life, so take your time! Do not get discouraged if you fall back or if you do not see the results as quickly as you would like. Once you get used to it, your inflammation will improve, and your great results will have you telling your doctor what helped with your success and you can share the good news with others.

Thanks for reading and happy anti-inflammatory dieting!

Finally, if you found this book useful in any way, a review on Amazon is always appreciated!